Oral Cancers

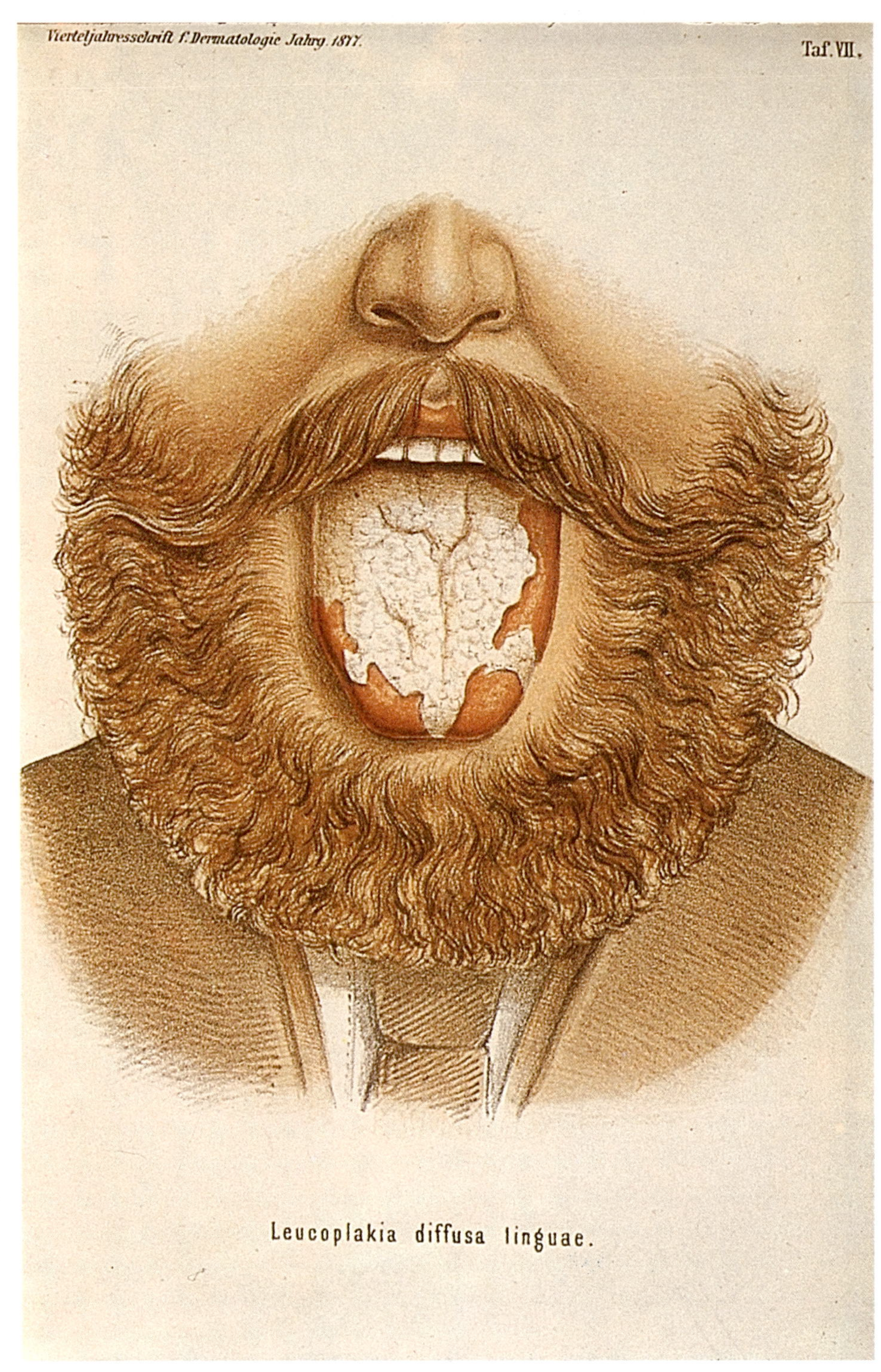

1 Extensive Leukoplakia of the mucosa of the tongue as originally illustrated by Ernst Schwimmer (1877).

A Colour Atlas of

Oral Cancers

The diagnosis and classification of leukoplakias, precancerous conditions and carcinomas

Priv. Doz. Dr. Med. Arne Burkhardt
Pathologisches Institut der Universität, Bern

Priv. Doz. Dr. Reinhard Maerker
Department of Oral and Maxillo-Facial Surgery
(Nordwestdeutsche Kieferklinik), University of Hamburg

Translated from the German by R.E.K. Meuss

Wolfe Medical Publications Ltd

Year Book Medical Publishers, Inc

Published by Wolfe Medical Publications Ltd, 1981
from the German edition, 'Vor-und Frühstadien des Mundhöhlenkarzinoms'
published by Carl Hanser Verlag.

Reprinted with minor amendments 1985

UK ISBN 0 7234 0769 X
US ISBN 0 8151 1337 4

Printed by Koesel GMBH & Co., Kempten/Allg.,
German Federal Republic.

General Editor, Wolfe Medical Atlases:
G Barry Carruthers, MD(London)

This book is one of the titles in the series of Wolfe Medical Atlases, a series which brings together probably the world's largest systematic published collection of diagnostic colour photographs.

Distributed in Continental North, South and Central America, Hawaii, Puerto Rico and The Philippines by
Year Book Medical Publishers, Inc.

For a full list of Atlases in the series, plus forthcoming titles and details of our surgical, dental and veterinary Atlases, please write to
Wolfe Medical Publications Ltd, Wolfe House,
3 Conway Street, London W1P 6HE
or
Year Book Medical Publishers, Inc,
35 East Wacker Drive, Chicago, Ill. 60601

Foreword

On a world-wide basis, the present phase of the fight against cancer is characterised by particular emphasis on certain subject areas. These include the detection and elimination or avoidance of risk factors in carcinogenesis, preventive measures (the diagnosis of precancerous or early stages of tumours in different organs), and improving the prognosis by starting optimum therapy as early as possible. A reduction in cancer mortality can be achieved only with greater interdisciplinary cooperation between specialists and general practitioners. This is also the aim of the many tumour centres opened in recent years, many of them also in the Federal Republic of Germany. They consider it one of their chief functions to develop optimum standardised treatment plans for the different forms of tumours.

Oral tumours are, in their precancerous and early stages, accessible to direct inspection. It was the great educational reformer Pestalozzi who said, 'Observation is the basis of all discoveries', and this holds true very particularly for the detection of oral cancer and its precancerous stages. The general practitioner and the dental surgeon thus carry the serious responsibility for recognising changes in the oral mucosa that may suggest cancer – the first stage in early diagnosis. The dental surgeon in particular plays a crucial role here, for he works within the oral cavity. In the same way, general practitioners, ENT specialists and dermatologists should make themselves thoroughly familiar with the appearance of early changes suggestive of carcinoma. Their knowledge and awareness is the precondition for the effective treatment of oral cancer which is mainly surgical and predominantly in the hands of oral and maxillo-facial surgeons.

The fuller diagnosis of such mucosal lesions generally calls for biopsy followed by pathohistological classification. Treatment is based on macroscopic as well as histological and cytological findings. Comparable statistics for treated cases from different hospitals will in their turn depend on the establishment of a uniform nomenclature and the staging and grading of tumours.

This colour atlas by A. Burkhardt and R. Maerker presents the results of years of fruitful cooperation between the Institute of Pathology and the North West German Hospital for Oral Diseases at the University of Hamburg. In 1978 the authors were awarded the Martini Prize for their researches in the field of precancerous and early stages of oral cancer. Colour photographs of the macroscopic appearance presenting on inspection of the mouth are shown facing the cellular substrate of the mucosal lesion. This, it is hoped, will train the eye of the physician and provide a better basis for the recognition of precancerous and early stages of oral cancer. To date research has established some fundamental principles relating to the genesis of oral carcinoma. These may be summed up as follows:

1 Oral cancer is 50 to 100 times more common in areas of the mucosa showing macroscopic changes than in those presenting an apparently normal appearance.
2 Dysplasia, i.e. cellular and tissue transformation in a previously normal mucosa, will as a rule precede malignant degeneration. A direct relationship exists between the degree of dysplasia and malignant degeneration.
3 The early stages of cancer tend to develop from multiple areas of dysplastic epithelium. In the same way, dysplastic areas are demonstrable in the vicinity of manifest carcinomas. Multiple preneoplasms thus point to field cancerisation.
4 Immunological reactions between tumour tissue and organism play a major role in the genesis, growth and spread of the tumours.

5 Surgical removal is the therapy of choice with precancerous lesions, as it has a positive effect on the prognosis for the early stages of cancer.

It is the aim of this colour atlas to improve the results that may be achieved in treating oral cancer, and therefore to reduce mortality. If this succeeds, it will reward years of concerted effort on the part of the authors and give great benefit to patients. Those being the aims, we hope the book will find wide acceptance among dentists and physicians, in particular ENT specialists, dermatologists, pathologists and oral surgeons.

Hamburg, spring 1981

Prof. G. Seifert, MD
Head of Institute of Pathology, The University of Hamburg.

Prof. G. Pfeifer, MD, DMD
Head of the Dept. for Oral and Dentofacial Surgery (North-West German Hospital for Oral Diseases) of the University Hospital for Dental and Oral Diseases in Hamburg.

Contents

Foreword 5

1 Introduction 9

2 The normal oral mucosa 13

3 Leukoplakia and precancerous lesions 23
- Definition and differentiation 23
  - (a) Leukoplakia 23
  - (b) Erythroplakia 24
- Clinical aspects of leukoplakia and erythroplakia 24
- Diagnostic procedure in leukoplakia and erythroplakia 26
- Histological examination 27
- Histological assessment and dysplasia classification 28
  - (a) Leukoplakias without or with only low-degree dysplasia 29
  - (b) Leukoplakias with a moderate degree of dysplasia 33
  - (c) Leukoplakias with a high degree of dysplasia and carcinoma *in situ* 33
  - (d) 'Candida leukoplakia' 34
- Clinical significance of the dysplasia classification – prognosis and treatment 34

4 Early stages of cancer and dissimulating cancers (carcinoma dissimulans) 81
- Clinical features 81
- Histopathology 81
- Therapy 83

5 Differential diagnosis 113
- White sponge naevus (naevus spongiosis albus mucosae) 113
- Smoker's palate (leukokeratosis nicotinica palati) 119
- Geographic tongue (lingua geographica, glossitis migrans) 125
- Median rhomboid glossitis (glossitis rhombica mediana) 129
- White changes in the mucosa arising from inflammatory lesions 135
- Non-malignant ulceration of the mucosa 141
- Mucosal changes associated with oral habits 151
- Fordyce spots (heterotopic sebaceous glands) 157
- Lichen planus 161
- Pemphigus vulgaris 171
- Dark pigmented patches (melanosis) 177

6 Bibliography 184

Index 185

1 Introduction

Inspection of the mouth forms part of every physical examination, as changes in the mucosa may be indicative of systemic disease. Infections, haematological, endocrine and dermatological conditions frequently produce characteristic changes in the mucosa while still at an early stage.

The oral mucosa must also be assessed for local conditions. Inflammatory lesions and keratosis as well as premalignant and malignant changes in the mucosa may be diagnosed on macroscopic inspection and palpation.

Experience has shown that there is insufficient general awareness of the opportunity offered by oral examination to diagnose premalignant lesions and the early stages of oral cancer, conditions which in Germany represent 2.5 per cent of manifest carcinomata. The oral cavity is open to inspection without recourse to surgical procedure; it provides ideal conditions for a simple, repeatable, low-cost routine check-up. Seventy per cent of carcinomata are more than 3cm in diameter by the time the patient comes for specialist treatment, a sign that precancerous lesions and the asymptomatic early stages of cancer are only rarely diagnosed by general practitioners. Thus an opportunity for effective treatment and a cure tends to be missed.

The early diagnosis and treatment of cancer are based on the concept that carcinomata develop over a long period of time, going through intermediate stages of different biological significance, and that treatment at this early or preinvasive stage offers the best prognosis and even the chance of a cure. This assumption has been proved correct by the positive results achieved in the field of gynaecology and gastroenterology.

The starting point for oral cancer is the mucosal epithelium. The oral cavity is the site where food is received, and therefore an area of the body where contact with exogenous material, micro-organisms and harmful agents is particularly intense. The oral mucosa functions as a mechanical as well as an immunological barrier. Contact with exogenous material means the likelihood of attack from micro-organisms (parasites, fungi, bacteria, viruses) on the one hand and exposure to microtraumata, irritants, toxins and carcinogens on the other. This includes direct traumatic lesions caused by food, alcohol, tobacco smoke, food toxins and carcinogens, and the metabolic products of the oral microflora, particularly where oral hygiene is poor, and also by mechanical and in some cases galvanic irritation from prostheses.

Protective mechanisms are an increased capacity for epithelial regeneration, and increased keratinisation which presents, on inspection, as leukoplakia, a white discoloration of the mucosa. These epithelial changes are reactive and reversible, but with progressive loss of normal control mechanisms they lead to precancerous states and oral carcinoma. Apart from the effects of contact with exogenous material, endogenous factors, such as genetic determination, hormonal factors, metabolic disease (*e.g.* iron deficiency, hepatic disease) also influence these changes.

Leukoplakia and oral cancer are more common in men than in women. Tobacco abuse and poor oral hygiene must be regarded as the principal risk factors arising from the Western European life style. The wide variety of damaging oral habits practised in developing countries play only a very minor role in this part of the world. These include the chewing of such materials as tobacco, betel nut (with or without the addition of slaked lime), coca leaves, spices, etc., and particularly smoking habits (burning end intraoral).

The term 'leukoplakia' has given rise to considerable misunderstanding since it was first defined more than 100 years ago by the dermatologist Ernst Schwimmer in 1877. The problem arises mainly because the term has been used partly as a clinical concept and partly as the histological diagnosis of a precancerous lesion. No uniform morphological substrate exists for the clinical diagnosis of leukoplakia, and only a proportion of clinically diagnosed leukoplakias represent true premalignant lesions. Histologically, the condition is based on a number of possible combinations of epithelial and stromal changes. These range from simple and harmless thickening of the epithelium (hyperplasia with hyperkeratosis), through precancerous epithelial dysplasia and carcinoma *in situ* to early invasive carcinoma.

Thanks to the work of Pindborg and his team in Denmark, the term leukoplakia is now used in reference to a purely clinical diagnosis relating to changes of varying biological significance, including the premalignant stages of oral cancer. The WHO Cancer Unit (1978) defines it as a white patch which is adherent to the mucosa and cannot be ascribed to any other condition. Distinction is made between pure white (homogeneous) leukoplakia, the precancerous nature of which is only facultative, and leukoplakia with reddish patches and erythroplakia (wholly red patches) which are regarded as precancerous lesions.

The decision as to whether these changes represent harmless epithelial changes (hyperplasia, inflammation), a genuinely precancerous condition or an early stage of manifest carcinoma, always has to be based on the histological examination of tissue obtained by biopsy or surgical excision.

Histological and cytological examination of sections under the microscope continues to be the basis on which differential diagnosis between precancerous conditions and early invasive carcinoma is made, despite the fact that a wide variety of far more sophisticated methods of investigation are now available (*e.g.* electron microscopy, exfoliative cytology, histochemistry, cytophotometry, cytogenic studies, clinical and immunological tests).

Cytological study of smear preparations taken from the oral mucosa is unlikely to play the same role in the diagnosis of premalignant and malignant changes in the oral cavity as it does at present in the field of gynaecology, because conditions for cell maturation are different. The lower part of the cervical canal presents a constantly migrating zone of epithelial transformation with fresh epithelial metaplasia and no marked keratinisation. The mouth, on the other hand, presents a fully mature stationary squamous epithelium with fully differentiated superficial cells which, as a rule, are maintained even over precancerous lesions. In general, it is unlikely that dysplastic cells from a deeper layer will be removed with a cytological smear. Biopsy of the oral mucosa, however, tends to be relatively uncomplicated and provide far more reliable information.

The term 'dysplasia' has proved useful in the differentiation of precancerous changes. It provides a measure of the degree of cell and tissue degeneration (slight, moderate, marked). Today the degree of dysplasia is used as the basis for a differential therapeutic approach in clinical medicine.

In large-scale studies of oral leukoplakia, 10 per cent of lesions have been found to show a marked degree of epithelial dysplasia and were considered to be genuine precancerous conditions. The same percentage of leukoplakias have been found to show actual degeneration.

Manifest, *i.e.* invasive, carcinoma may, in fact, be masked for a considerable time by nonspecific macroscopic changes, such as leukoplakic alterations in the mucosa, ulceration and papillomatous growths.

The broad spectrum of changes occurring in the oral mucosa has been excellently described in a number of books and atlases by such competent authors as Strassburg and Knolle, Tyldesley, and Pindborg. Not enough attention has been paid, however, to the very important subject of early cancer diagnosis.

This Atlas sets out to show the importance of macroscopic inspection of the mouth in clinical practice and what can be achieved by it, in conjunction with histological studies.

There is urgent need for greater awareness in this area, not only as part of a general medical examination, but in the course of specialist examinations by dentists, oral dentofacial and plastic surgeons, ENT specialists and dermatologists. The Atlas is intended to aid clinical assessment and, by including the histological features, to provide greater insight into the way in which the pathological diagnosis is made. Conversely, it is, of course, essential for pathologists to know the clinical features in this field and be conversant with the clinical problems involved.

The Atlas is designed for everyday practical use, and for this reason historical and theoretical aspects of oral cancer have been deliberately omitted. A bibliography is included, where references may be readily found. The Atlas is based on many years of close collaboration between a clinician and a pathologist in an endeavour to improve the early diagnosis of cancer.

Where detailed data are given, these are based on the histological examination of 906 biopsies from oral leukoplakias and precancerous changes and 1,294 biopsies from oral carcinomata, and on a retrospective clinical and pathological study of 200 patients with leukoplakia, the average period of observation being $5\frac{1}{2}$ years. Full details of the results are given elsewhere.

Corresponding clinical and histological illustrations are shown on facing pages for ease of comparison. In each case the clinical and histological diagnoses are given as a heading. Clinical management and suggestions for treatment are also included.

2 The normal oral mucosa

Knowledge of normal conditions is the prerequisite for diagnosis of pathological changes. The normal mucosa presents a moist, glistening surface, and is a rose or greyish-pink colour due to the vascular bed in the connective tissue underlying the epithelium being well supplied with blood. The movability of the oral mucosa varies, and distinction is made between locolabile (lip, cheek, tongue, floor of mouth) and locostable (hard palate, gums) areas (Table 1).

Table 1 Histological Structure of the Oral Mucosa

	Locolabile mucosa	Locostable mucosa
Stratified epithelium		
Basal layer	+	+
Prickle-cell layer	+	+
Granular layer	–	+/(+)
Horny layer	+	+/++
Orthokeratosis (anucleate)	–	+
Parakeratosis (nucleate)	+	–
Rete pegs/connective tissue papillae	shallow	deep
Lamina propria	wide, loose	narrow, fibrous
Occurrence	lip, cheek, tongue, floor of mouth	palate, gingiva

Histological examination shows the surface to be covered with a stratified squamous epithelium, with the sequence of layers similar to that seen in the epidermis of the skin. A basal cell layer (stratum basale), spinous layer (stratum spinosum) and flattened horny layer (stratum corneum) may be distinguished. A granular layer (stratum granulosum) is found only in areas showing orthokeratotic keratinisation. However, as a rule, there is clearly less keratinisation than in the epidermis. Differentiation is made between orthokeratosis, with a granular layer and anucleated squames, and parakeratosis, with nucleated squames. The degree and type of keratinisation show considerable variation (Table 1). In areas not subject to much mechanical stress, such as the cheek, parakeratosis is frequently only demonstrable with special staining techniques, while areas subject to mechanical stress, such as the gums and the hard palate, show orthokeratosis like the epidermis. Particular structural elements in the epithelium are the attachment plaques, or desmosomes. These provide mechanical intercellular cohesion and are responsible for the appearance of 'prickle' cells. The tonofibrils, which act as an 'internal skeleton', and the keratin produced from them afford mechanical protection. Their quantity and density determine the translucency of the epithelial layer and hence the macroscopic coloration of the mucosa. Increased keratinisation, as in the epithelial hyperplasia known as leukoplakia and in hyperkeratosis, causes the rosy tinge of the mucosa to give way to the naturally whitish colour of the epithelium. Decreased keratinisation, *e.g.* in dysplastic epithelial atrophy, causes dark red discoloration of the mucosa (erythroplakia).

The interdigitation of epithelium (rete pegs) and connective tissue (papillae) also shows considerable variation, being more marked in areas subject to greater wear and tear. The subepithelial connective tissue contains a dense network of capillaries that supply it with blood, and is richly innervated. The muscularis mucosae, which in other mucous membranes separates the lamina propria from the underlying connective tissue, is absent.

Both the epithelium and subepithelial tissues contain cells with nonspecific defensive functions (leukocytes) and immunocompetent cells conferring local immunity (lymphocytes and plasma cells in subepithelial tissues; lymphocytes, cerebriform lymphoid cells and Langerhans' cells in the epithelium). The special features of lymphoepithelial symbiosis in the region of the tonsillar ring need not be considered here.

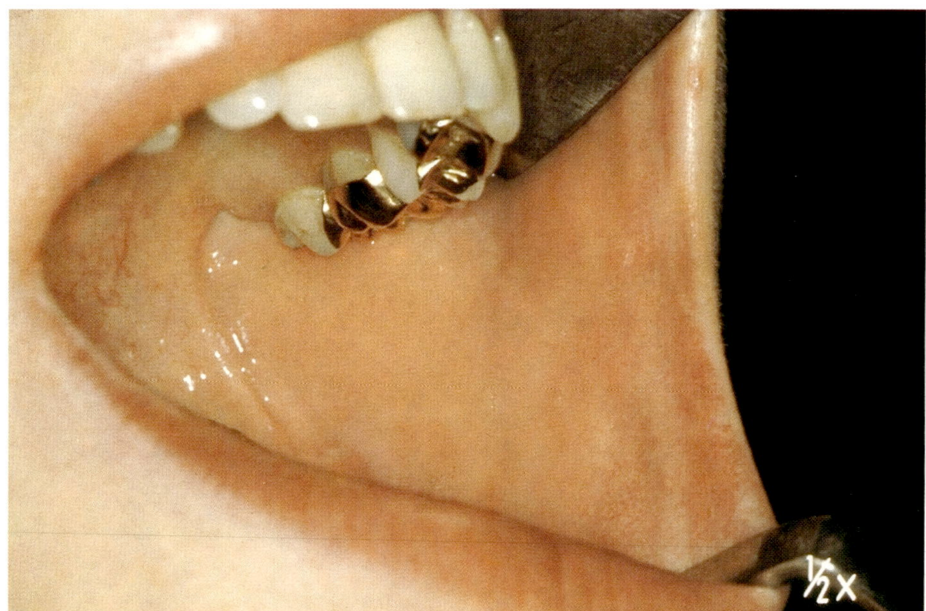

2

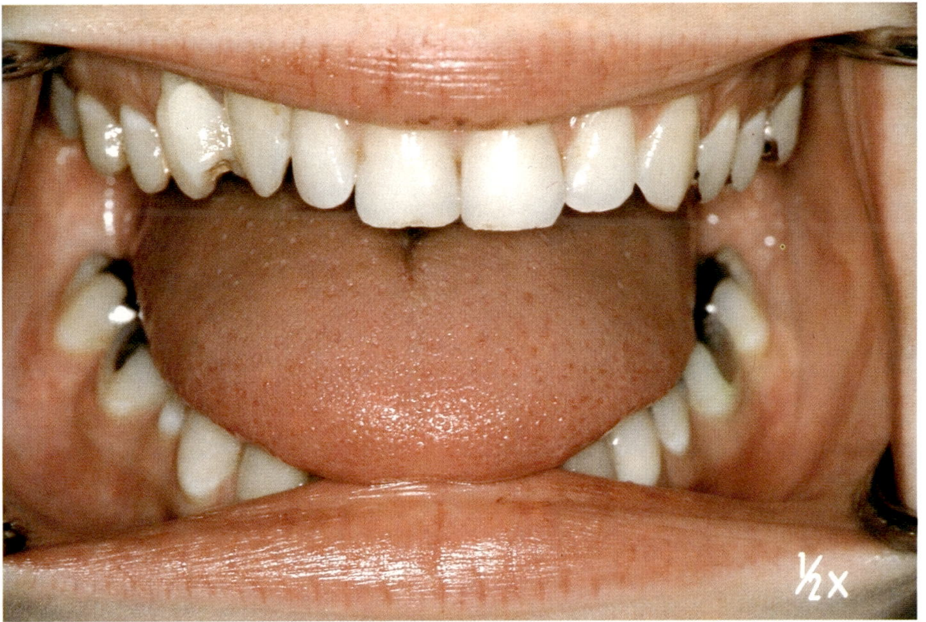

3

2 **Mucosa of the left cheek and maxilla,** pale pink, moist and shiny. (Female patient aged 20)

3 **Normal mucosa of tongue** Superior surface is moist, showing normal appearance. (Female patient aged 20)

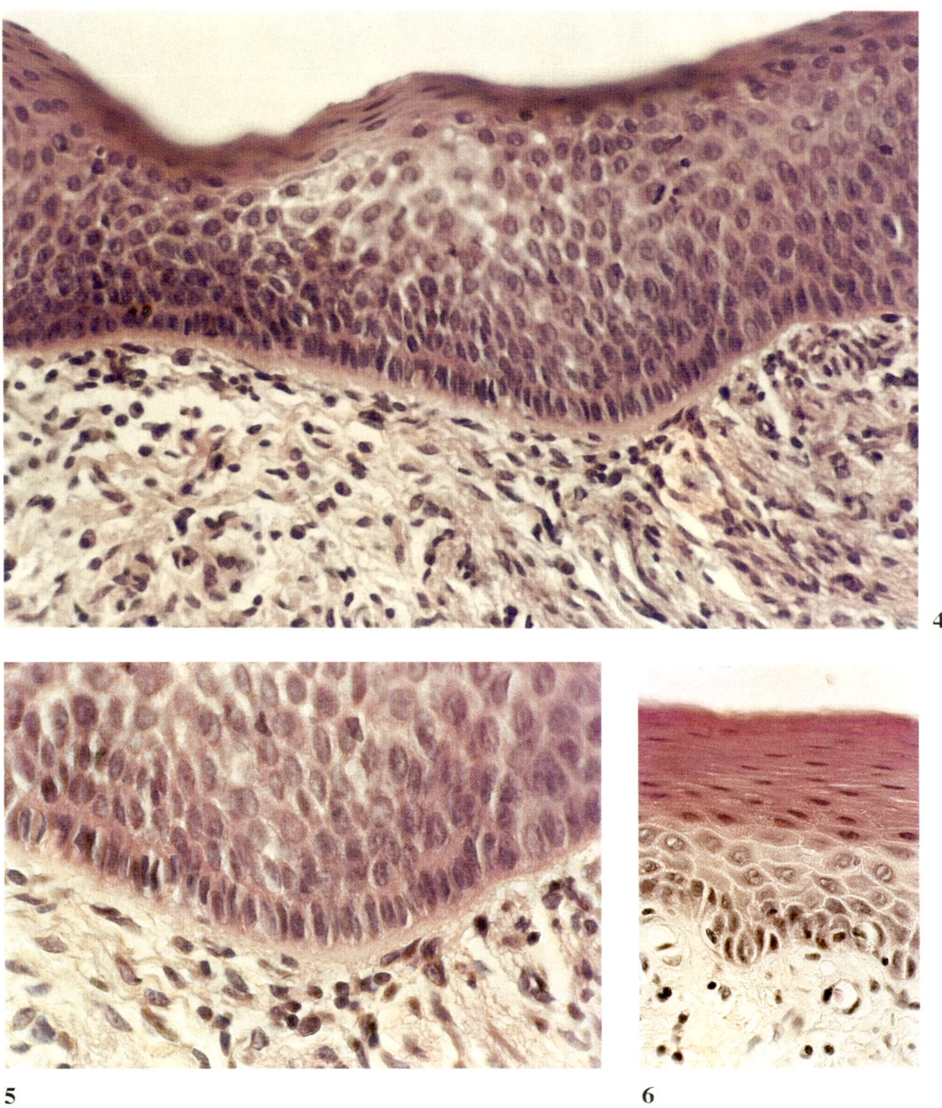

4

5 6

4 Normal mucosa of the cheek Epithelium with wave-like rete pegs only just discernible and there is no more marked interdigitation of epithelium and connective tissue. Basal layer is clearly delineated with cells polar. Above it lies a narrow spinous layer and superficial to this, are flattened keratinised squames which have retained their nuclei (parakeratosis). Below the epithelium, loosely structured connective tissue shows vessels and occasional inflammatory cells.

5 Greater magnification clearly shows the cells of the basal layer at right angles to the epithelial–mesenchymal interface, forming a single cell layer. Superficial to these are regular 'prickle' cells and between them occasional interepithelial cells.

6 Mucosa of the cheek Special staining demonstrates keratinisation (keratin appears red). It is apparent that keratinisation starts in the middle spinous layer. *(Chesa)*

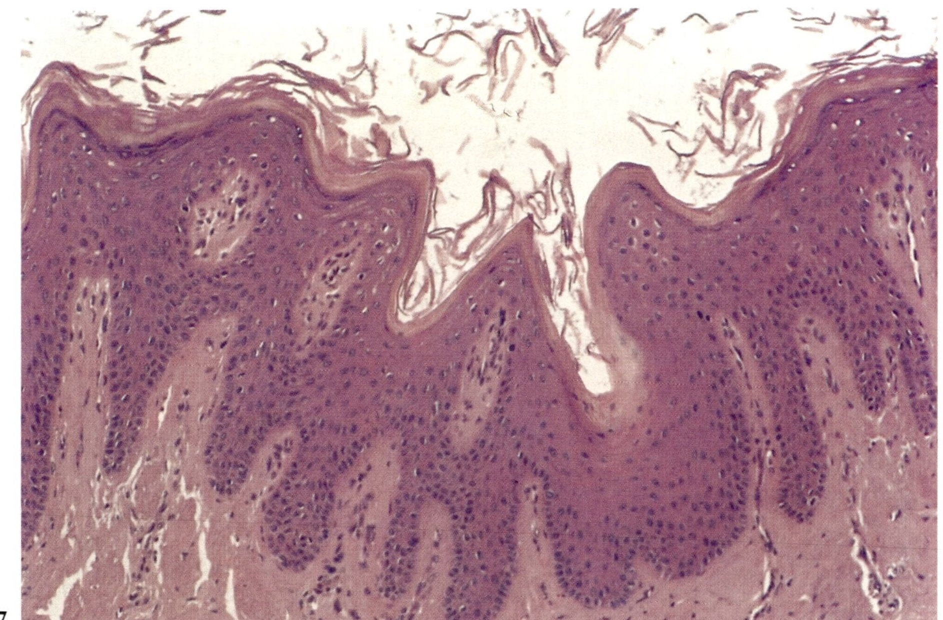

7

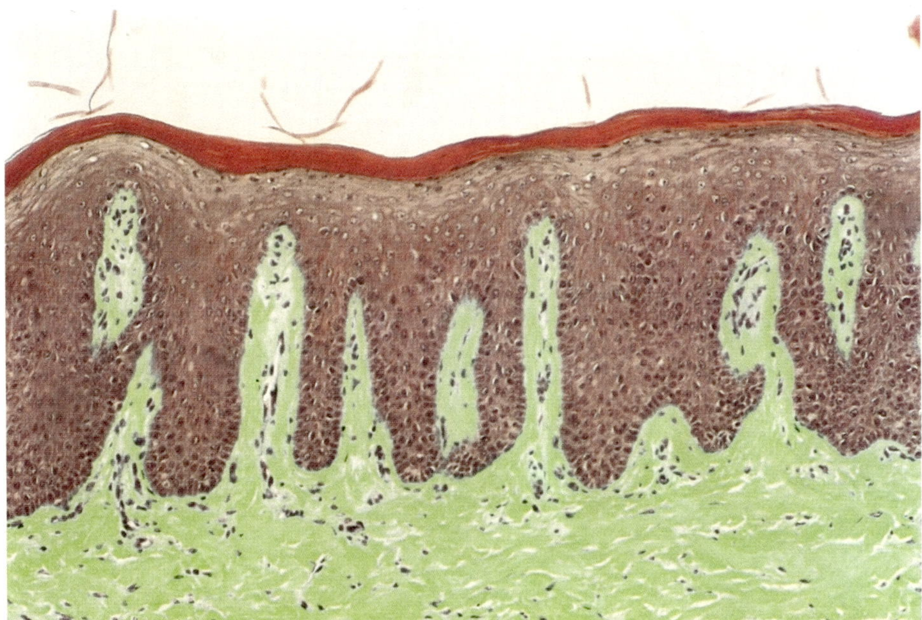

8

7 Mucosa of hard palate Rete pegs are numerous, deep and slender, and extend from the epithelium into the connective tissue. Interdigitation of epithelium and mesenchyme is therefore quite marked. Superficially are a narrow granular layer, not easily discernible at this magnification, and lamellar keratinised squames with no trace of nuclei (orthokeratosis).

8 Normal mucosa of the palate Masson–Goldner stain has produced green coloration of subepithelial connective tissue. Superficially, the red, anucleated keratinised layer stands out clearly. *(Masson–Goldner)*

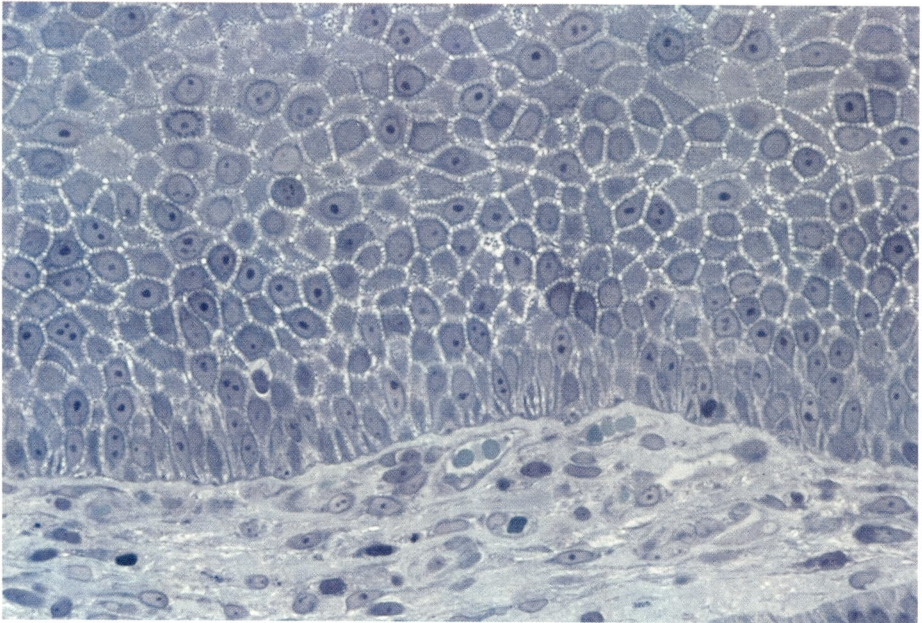

9

9 Semi-thin section of normal oral mucosa (floor of mouth) Basal cells are clearly polar in arrangement. Above them is a spinous layer with desmosomes projecting and forming a circle of 'prickles' around the cells. *(Toluidine blue)*

10 (top) Basal cells The elongated oval nuclei (N) are polar and lie perpendicular to the epithelial–mesenchymal interface. Nuclei contain little heterochromatin and small nucleoli. Mitochondria and occasional bundles of tonofibrils can be seen. The bases of the cells are delineated by the narrow 'electron-microscopic' basal membrane. (Str = stroma; × 8,000)

10 (below) High magnification of epithelial–mesenchymal interface The meandering line of the 'electron microscopic' basal membrane (*Star*) is clearly discernible. Superficial to it are intracellular bundles of tonofibrils (T). Deeper down, in the mesenchyme, are typical collagen fibrils (K). (× 16,800)

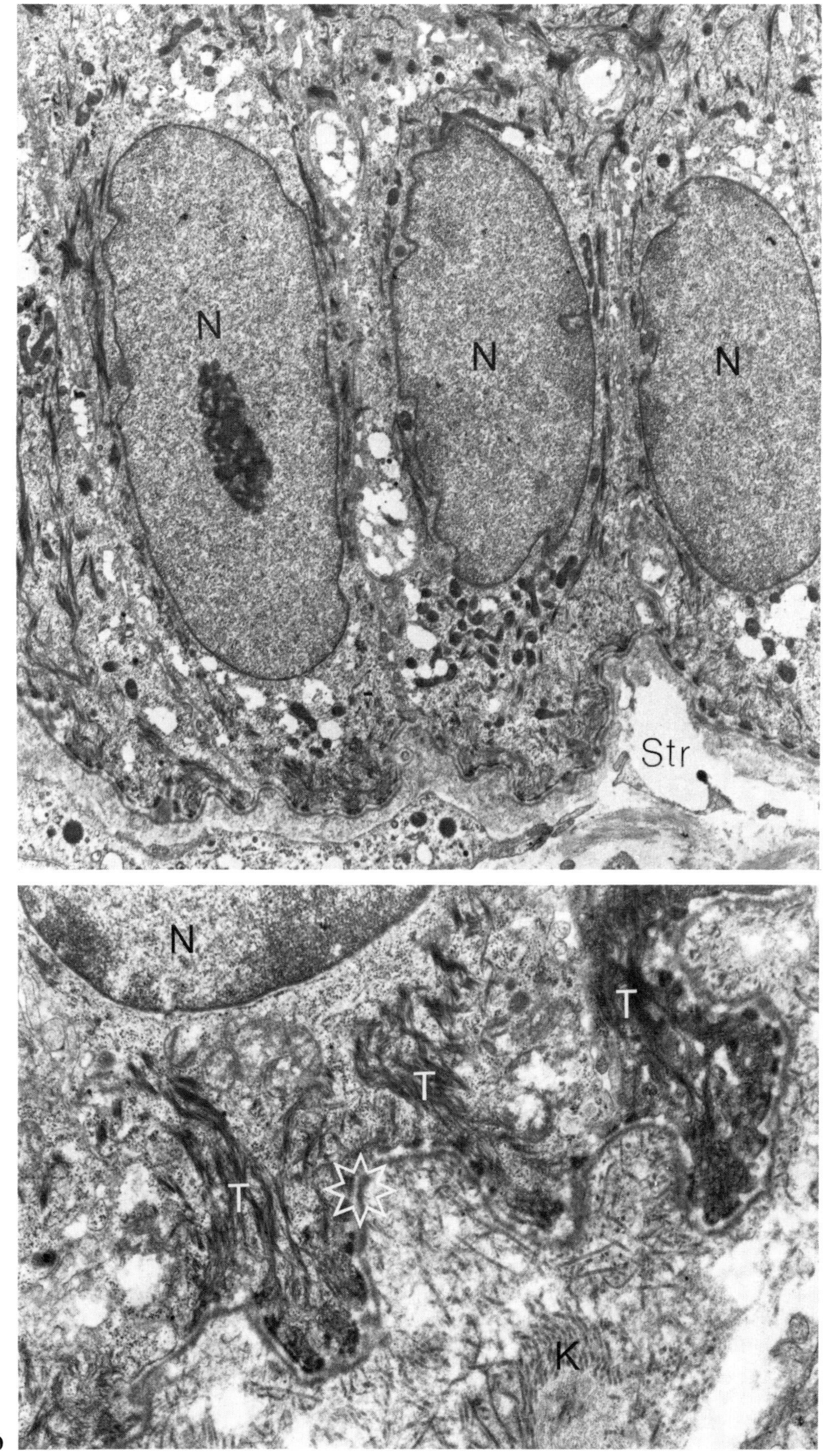

10

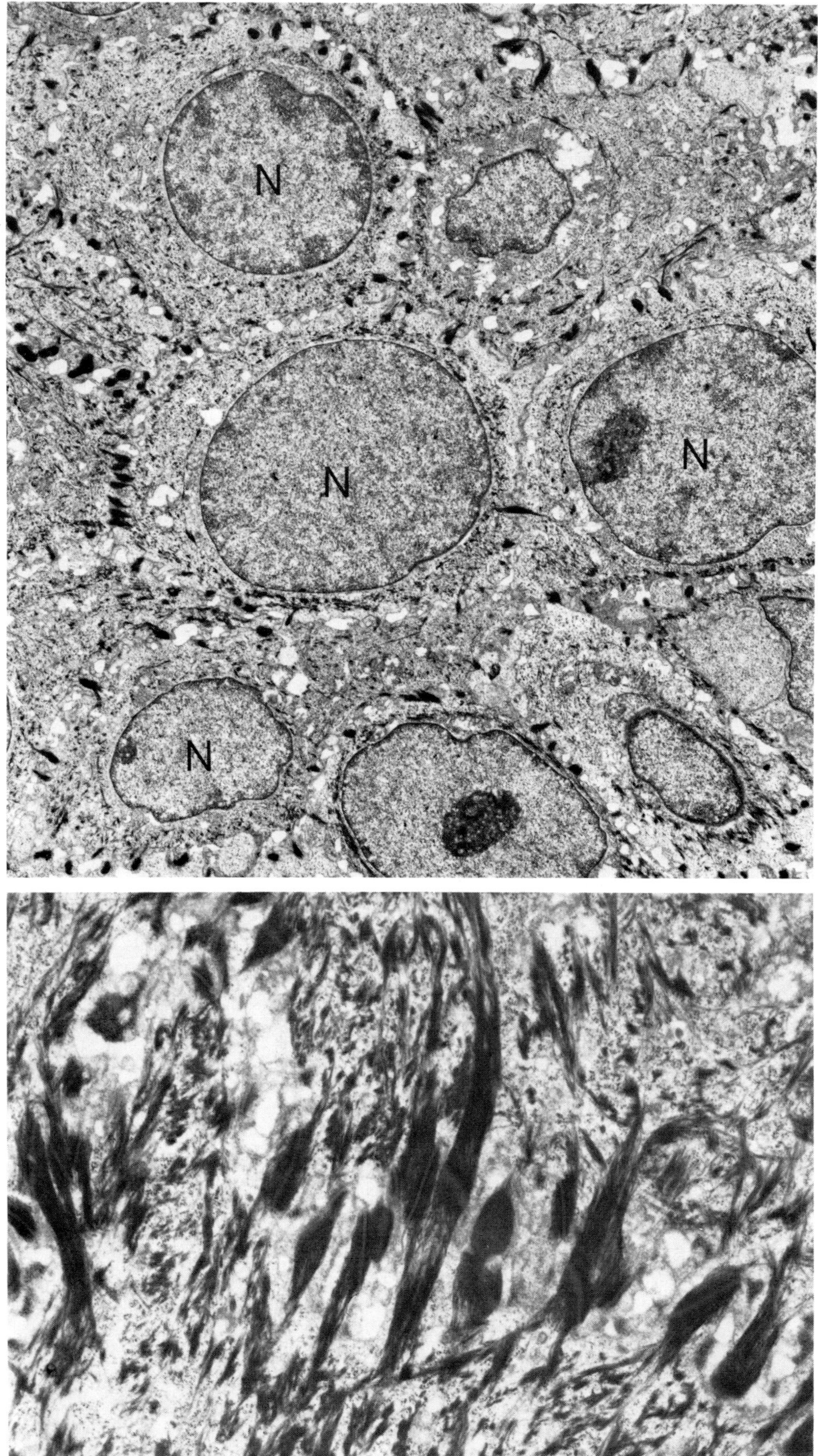

11

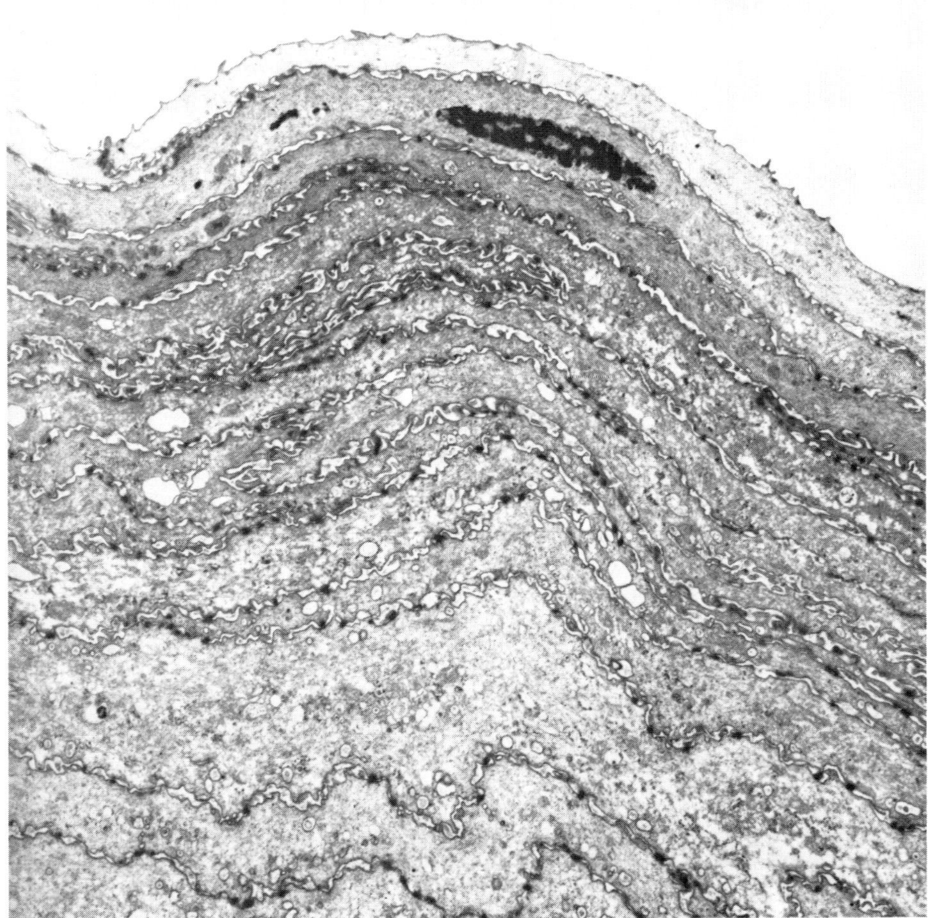

12

11 (top) Prickle cells (electron micrograph) Large nuclei, oval and rounded (N), containing little heterochromatin and small nucleoli. In the cytoplasm, only a few fine tonofibril bundles are seen. Desmosomes stand out clearly in the region of the plasma membranes. (× 4,800)

11 (below) Plasma membranes highly magnified to show linear desmosomes and relatively dense tonofibril bundles running down to them. (× 15,900)

12 The superficial horny layer (electron micrograph) The membrane enclosing the keratinised squames, which are several deep, stands out clearly. Remnants of nuclei are clearly discernible in one place (parakeratosis). (× 4,800)

3 Leukoplakia and precancerous lesions

Precancerous lesions are tissue changes more frequently found to undergo malignant degeneration than normal tissue of the same type. In the oral mucosa they present as the whitish lesions of leukoplakia and the reddish lesions of erythroplakia. Another form, speckled or nodular leukoplakia, is a mixture of leukoplakia and erythroplakia which is classified as a leukoplakia (see page 24).

Definition and differentiation

a) Leukoplakia

Leukoplakia is defined as a white patch on the mucosa that cannot be rubbed off and is not ascribable to any other condition (Cancer Unit of the World Health Organisation). The diagnosis is therefore descriptive, with no aetiological definition and a negative differentiation from other conditions. All known conditions also presenting with whitish changes in the mucosa, such as lichen planus and leukokeratosis nicotinica, need to be excluded (see Chapter 5). Not every whitish patch in the mouth is leukoplakia, and, of course, not every leukoplakia is a precancer.

The aetiological classification established by Schürmann, Greither and Hornstein is of value in that it induces the clinician not to stop at the diagnosis of leukoplakia, but to look for systemic and local causes (Table 2). Differentiation is made between:

1 Hereditary and idiopathic leukoplakias.
2 Endogenous irritative leukoplakias (with inflammatory and dermatological conditions).
3 Exogenous irritative leukoplakias (poorly fitting dentures, tobacco abuse, etc.).

The first two forms tend to be harmless, requiring either no treatment at all or treatment in conjunction with the underlying condition. Exogenous irritative aetiology needs to be excluded if macroscopic inspection of the leukoplakia does not suggest carcinoma (see below). After exclusion of harmful factors (correction of new dentures, dental treatment as required, the use of compatible metals, strict oral hygiene, stopping tobacco abuse) and conservative treatment, one may at the least expect an improvement in the condition. It is therefore necessary to keep the lesion under observation for a time. Clinical experience has shown that a large proportion of these leukoplakias tend to become autonomous and therefore will not respond to this form of treatment. Such lesions urgently require further investigation and specialist treatment. Histological examination is normally required, with further treatment dependent on the findings.

Table 2 Aetiological Factors in Oral Precancer and Cancer

Exogenous	Endogenous
Tobacco	Hereditary factors
Alcohol	Liver disease
Particular oral habits (morsicatio buccarum, chewing tobacco, betel nut)	Malnutrition (Vitamin/protein deficiency)
	Iron deficiency
Poor oral hygiene	Diabetes mellitus
Food particles	Hormonal factors
Bacterial products	Systemic infection (syphilis)
Local infection (herpes virus, Candica albicans)	
Irritation from dentures	
Galvanic irritation	
Exposure to toxins	
(lead, mercury, benzol)	

These 'facultative' precancers are the problem leukoplakias. They may be defined as a white patch in the mucosa, that cannot be rubbed off and is not ascribable to any other disease, and whose further existence no longer depends on the continued harmful effects of the putative triggering factors (autonomous behaviour).

b) Erythroplakia

Erythroplakia is defined as a brilliant, dark-red circumscribed lesion that cannot be rubbed off and is not ascribable to any other definitive condition. The margin of such a lesion may also show whitish (leukoplakic) changes. Erythroplakia is less common than leukoplakia and has, on the whole, greater malignant potential. Erythroplakic lesions frequently overlie oral cancers that are in their early stages.

Clinical aspects of leukoplakia and erythroplakia

Leukoplakic lesions do not present a uniform appearance with regard to colour and surface configuration, and distinction may be made between entirely white (homogeneous) and patchy, often verrucoid forms (Table 3). The latter develop as a mixture of leukoplakic and erythroplakic areas. The following classification into three forms has proved useful (Table 4):

1 Simple leukoplakia
2 Verrucous leukoplakia
3 Erosive leukoplakia

This classification immediately provides the clinician with a rough idea about the significance of the lesion and hence its prognosis (Table 5). *Simple leukoplakia*, the purely white form, is quite common and considered the most benign. Malignant degeneration is likely to occur in only three per cent of cases where the condition has persisted for some time. *Verrucous leukoplakia* holds an intermediate position, but

Table 3 Macroscopic Clinical Forms of Leukoplakia. Comparison of Pindborg classification with that of Bánóczy and Sugár

Homogeneous leukoplakia	Leukoplakia simplex
	Leukoplakia verrucosa
Patchy leukoplakia	Leukoplakia erosiva

Table 4 Oral Leukoplakias. Macroscopic Clinical Classification

Leukoplakia	Characteristics
Leukoplakia simplex	Whiteness homogeneous, clearly circumscribed, surface smooth or slightly undulating and granular 49% of all leukoplakias Rarely precancerous
Leucoplakia verrucosa	Irregular, nodular surface Slightly patchy, greyish red 27% of all leukoplakias
Leukoplakia erosiva	Irregular surface Very patchy, with erosions 24% of all leukoplakias Rate of malignant degeneration 38%

Table 5 Macroscopic Clinical Forms of Oral Leukoplakia and their Clinical Progress (%; n = 200 patients)

	Leukoplakia simplex (n = 98)	Leukoplakia verrucosa (n = 54)	Leukoplakia erosiva (n = 48)
No recurrence	71	61	46
Improvement	13	18	6
No change	5	4	6
Recurrence	8	6	4
Carcinoma	3	11	38

clinically it must always be regarded with suspicion. *Erosive leukoplakia* always rates as a high-risk condition, with up to 38 per cent later showing malignant degeneration, *i.e.* it carries the highest percentage of genuinely precancerous lesions. An even higher percentage is found, however, among the relatively uncommon pure erythroplakias.

The prognosis in leukoplakia also depends on the localisation of the lesion and the age of the patient. With leukoplakias of the palate or alveolar ridge, malignant transformation is relatively uncommon and their removal is not usually followed by recurrence. Any cancers found on the alveolar ridge have probably developed without a preliminary leukoplakic stage. Leukoplakias on the floor of the mouth and at the root of the tongue, on the other hand, will much more frequently show transition to invasive growth. Verrucous and erosive leukoplakias are less commonly found in the area of the root of the tongue, with invasive carcinomata relatively more frequent, and it must be assumed that malignant transformation is particularly rapid in this area, with omission of some preliminary stages. If verrucous or erosive changes are found on clinical examination, histological studies will usually show an early invasive carcinoma. A possible explanation could be that the floor of the mouth is the 'drainage' area of the oral cavity where carcinogenic substances collect and remain for longer periods. The floor of the mouth and the margin of the tongue must therefore be considered areas of particular risk.

The peak age of incidence for leukoplakia lies beyond the 50th year, and malignant development also increases with age. The sex distribution shows a predisposition towards men (1.3:1), and the rate of malignant degeneration is also nearly twice as great in males as in females. Dental restorations in conjunction with poor oral hygiene and badly fitting prostheses, alcohol and tobacco abuse are potential irritant and risk-factors and may have an unfavourable effect on subsequent development. Denture-wearers frequently also show *Candida albicans* populations (see page 34).

Erythroplakias are not subdivided on the basis of their clinical appearance. The marginal zones of the homogeneously red area in the mucosa frequently show minor whitish changes. If the leukoplakic component is of large extent, the lesion is traditionally referred to as 'patchy leukoplakia' (verrucous or erosive leukoplakia); the term 'patchy erythroplakia' would be equally justifiable but is not normally used.

Diagnostic procedure in leukoplakia and erythroplakia

With leukoplakias and erythroplakias of the oral cavity, the methods of diagnosis will depend on the individual situation, with account being taken of the factors discussed above. The diagram opposite provides a general guide.

Biopsies should be obtained from any leukoplakia that persists or looks suspicious. Erythroplakia always calls for biopsy, and if located in the region of the floor or tongue the patient must be admitted to hospital and a fast-frozen section made. In principle, it is possible to remove only a small representative part of the mucosal lesion (biopsy), or to remove the whole area that has shown mucosal changes from the beginning (excision). Excision is always preferable if the lesion is not too extensive and the location presents no technical problems. Where there are clinical grounds to suspect cancer, malignancy should first be excluded or confirmed by biopsy and frozen section so that radical surgery, if necessary, may be performed immediately. The biological significance of the lesion can only be established by histological examination, and this will then determine the further course of treatment (see below).

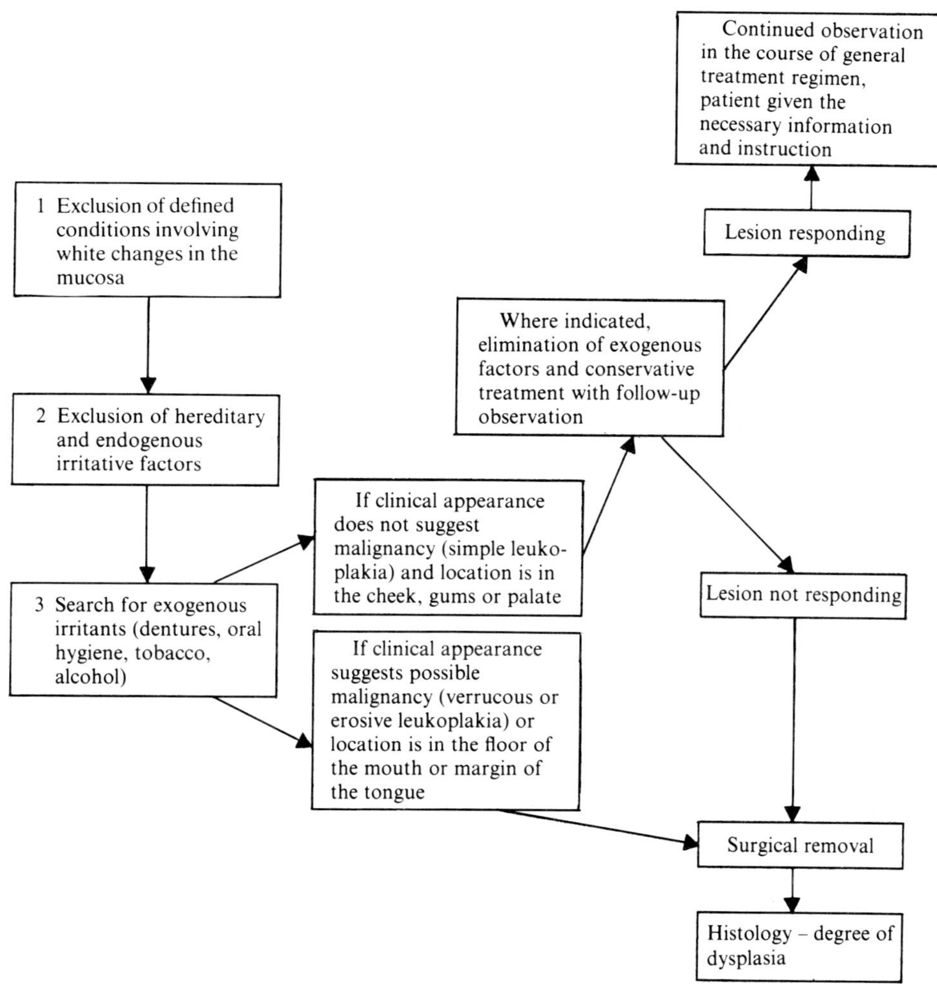

Histological examination

If invasive diagnosis (biopsy or excision) is decided upon, it is necessary to make sure that the removed tissue is given optimum preparation and evaluation. A full and reliable diagnosis and consequently correct treatment will depend on this.

Biopsies should not be too small, therefore, as small pieces of epithelial tissue permit only limited assessment, and it is also possible that the material may not be properly embedded or sections may be cut at the wrong angle. The piece of tissue should be approx. 1 × 0.5cm in area, so that it can still be cut longitudinally after fixation. Larger areas of excised mucosa should be attached to cork plates for fixation. Care must be taken not to crush the material or force it into too small a container. Fixation needs to be done immediately, ideally in freshly made up Bouin's solution (saturated picric acid

1.2 per cent, formaldehyde 40 per cent, and glacial acetic acid, in proportions of 15:5:1), as this will also permit immunohistological studies on the embedded material. For everyday use, a 4 per cent formalin solution adequately serves as a fixative.

After fixation the tissue is cut to size. Small biopsy specimens are cut in half lengthwise, while larger pieces obtained by excision are divided into narrow parallel strips (2–3mm in width). The proposed line of section should be colour-marked, to avoid cutting into previously adjacent surfaces. Where large amounts of tissue have been surgically removed, it will, of course, be possible only to examine carefully selected representative areas. If size permits, a complete cross-section of the lesion should be produced so that the margins of excision, the transition from normal to diseased mucosa and the central lesion can be clearly assessed.

The material is embedded in paraffin by the usual method, taking particular care with the positioning of the tissue within the block, using a stereomicroscope, if necessary. Sections must be cut exactly vertical to the surface of the mucosa, giving an orthograde section of the epithelium. This permits accurate assessment of the rete pegs and any invasive growth.

The tissue sections must be stained in every case with haematoxylin and eosin as well as periodic acid–Schiff (PAS). The PAS reaction stains the 'light-microscopic' basement membrane and subepithelial Russell bodies and clearly demonstrates fungal growth. Masson–Goldner staining will, in addition, provide selective coloration of connective tissue (green) and keratin (red) to facilitate assessment of normal and pathological keratinisation. For routine purposes, special keratin staining (Chesa) may be omitted and the use of silver to identify the basement membrane is necessary only in exceptional cases.

For specific questions, particularly the differential diagnosis of dermatological conditions, immunohistological demonstration of various proteins, particularly immunoglobulins, may provide important diagnostic information. The indirect immunoperoxidase method permits this to be done even with material already embedded in paraffin (Löning et al. 1977).

Histological assessment and dysplasia classification

Histological examination determines first of all whether the lesion has already become an invasive carcinoma or is still benign. Benign lesions need to be further differentiated, however, as they may be harmless epithelial hyperplasias, but can also be associated with epithelial changes that must be regarded precancerous. The *degree of dysplasia* is therefore determined as a measure of tissue and cellular deviation from the norm (Table 6).

Table 6 Histological Characteristics of Epithelial Hyperplasia and Epithelial Dysplasia

Characteristics of epithelial hyperplasia	Characteristics of epithelial dysplasia
Hyperkeratosis	Basal cell hyperplasia
Orthokeratosis	Loss of basal cell polarity
Parakeratosis	Cellular polymorphism
Acanthosis	Increased rate of mitosis
Leukoedema	Dyskeratosis
Spongiosis	Epithelial stratification abnormal

Studies in the field of clinical pathology have clearly shown that moderate and, particularly, high degrees of epithelial dysplasia carry an increased risk of carcinomatous development. The degree of dysplasia thus provides the key criterion for determining the prognosis and deciding on the most effective form of treatment (see page 34).

The diagnosis and classification of dysplasia are based on six relevant histological and cytological parameters (Table 6). These are changes in the basal cell layer as an indication of increased proliferative kinetics in the region, changes in the appearance of individual cells, an increase in mitotic figures, and abnormal keratinisation of individual cells in the prickle cell layer (dyskeratosis, Figure **15**). Abnormal and absent epithelial stratification are the final stages of a progressive epithelial degeneration that is highly characteristic of carcinoma *in situ* (see page 33). This dysplasia classification applies not only to leukoplakia but also to erythroplakia.

Additional indicators for dysplasia are an increase in subepithelial lymphocytes, plasma cells and interepithelial cells ('stroma reaction'), and the presence of *Candida* organisms.

The ultrastructure also shows characteristic changes due to leukoplakia with or without dysplasia. Leukoplakia *without* dysplasia shows enhanced tissue differentiation (prosoplasia) with an increase in tissue-specific elements (tonofibrils, desmosomes). The basement membrane may be doubled, indicating enhanced cell regeneration. Leukoplakia *with* dysplasia also shows ultrastructural tissue degeneration (anaplasia), which takes the form of both quantitative and qualitative changes in structural elements. The desmosomes are reduced in number and simpler in construction, cellular cohesion and communication are disrupted. Tonofibrils are not inserted into desmosomes, so that their architectural configuration is abnormal, and perinuclear clumping, spiral formation and cell necrosis are seen (dyskeratosis, dyskeratotic necrosis). The basement membrane is thin and shows gaps, and the cell membranes of basal cells may show microinvasion in these areas.

a) Leukoplakias without or with only low-degree dysplasia

With this form of leukoplakia, the parameters for epithelial hyperplasia show variation in degree (Table 6). The whitish hypertrophy of the mucosa is due to increased keratinisation (hyperkeratosis) at the surface and thickening of the prickle cell layer (acanthosis) beneath. Mucosal keratinisation may take the form of anucleate horny squames (orthokeratosis) or of remnants of nuclei persisting in the keratinocytes (parakeratosis). Less common features are cells swollen with intracellular water or oedematous enlargement of intercellular spaces (leukoedema, ballooning, spongiosis).

These leukoplakias are generally planar, with exophytic and endophytic forms relatively uncommon. They thus correspond largely to simple leukoplakia. It has been found practicable to include lesions with no signs of dysplasia and those with minor dysplastic changes in one group, as low-degree dysplasia may also represent a completely harmless reversible epithelial irritation. This group of harmless leukoplakias is not to be considered precancerous and, accounting for 74 per cent, represents the majority of oral leukoplakias.

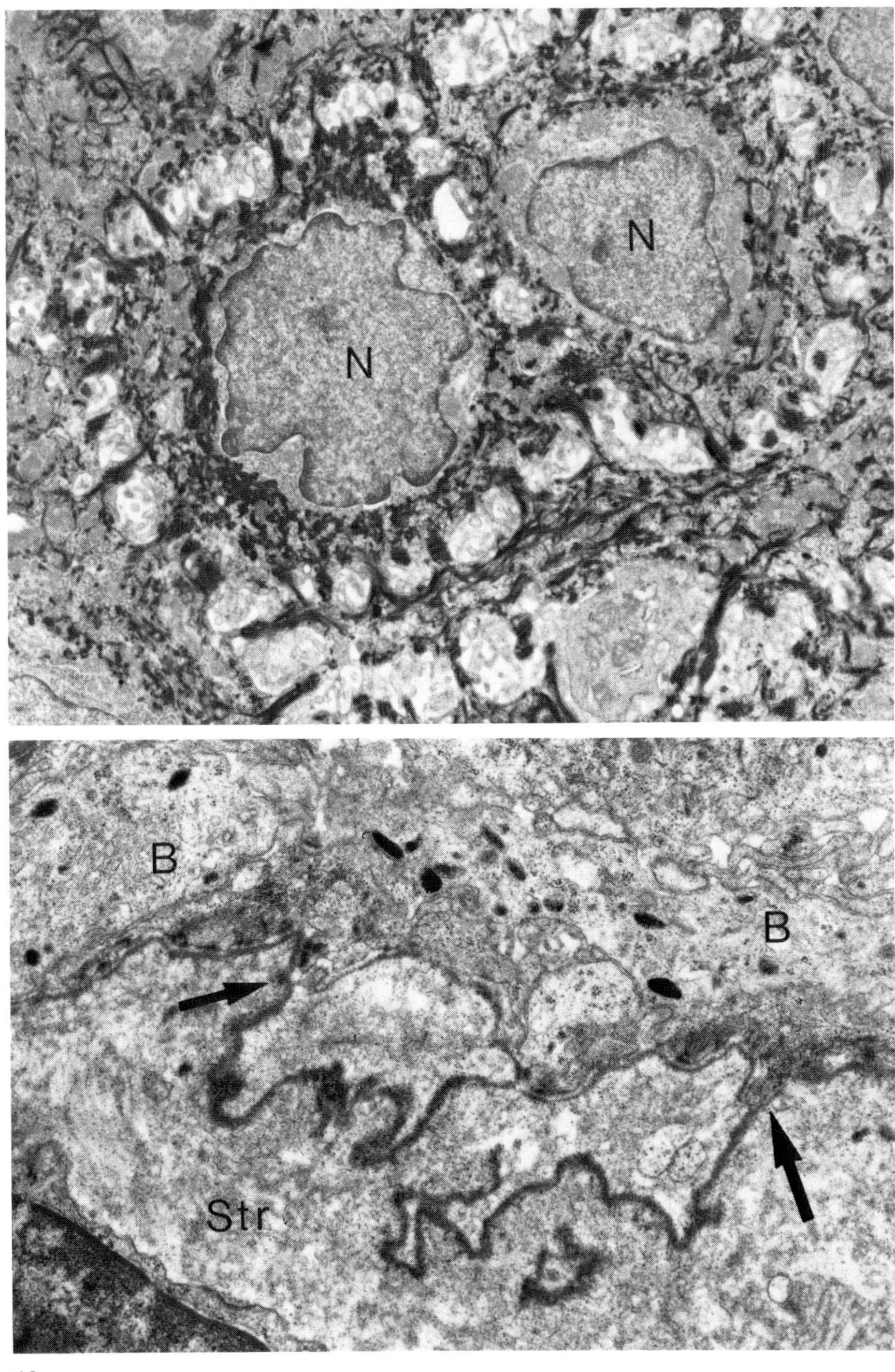

13

13 (top) **Prickle cells** showing a marked increase and thickening of tonofibril bundles. Desmosomal cell connections are well established. (N = nuclei; × 7,800)

13 (below) Partial detachment of basement membrane *(between arrows)* with formation of narrow new basement membrane. (B = basal cell, Str = stroma; × 15,600)

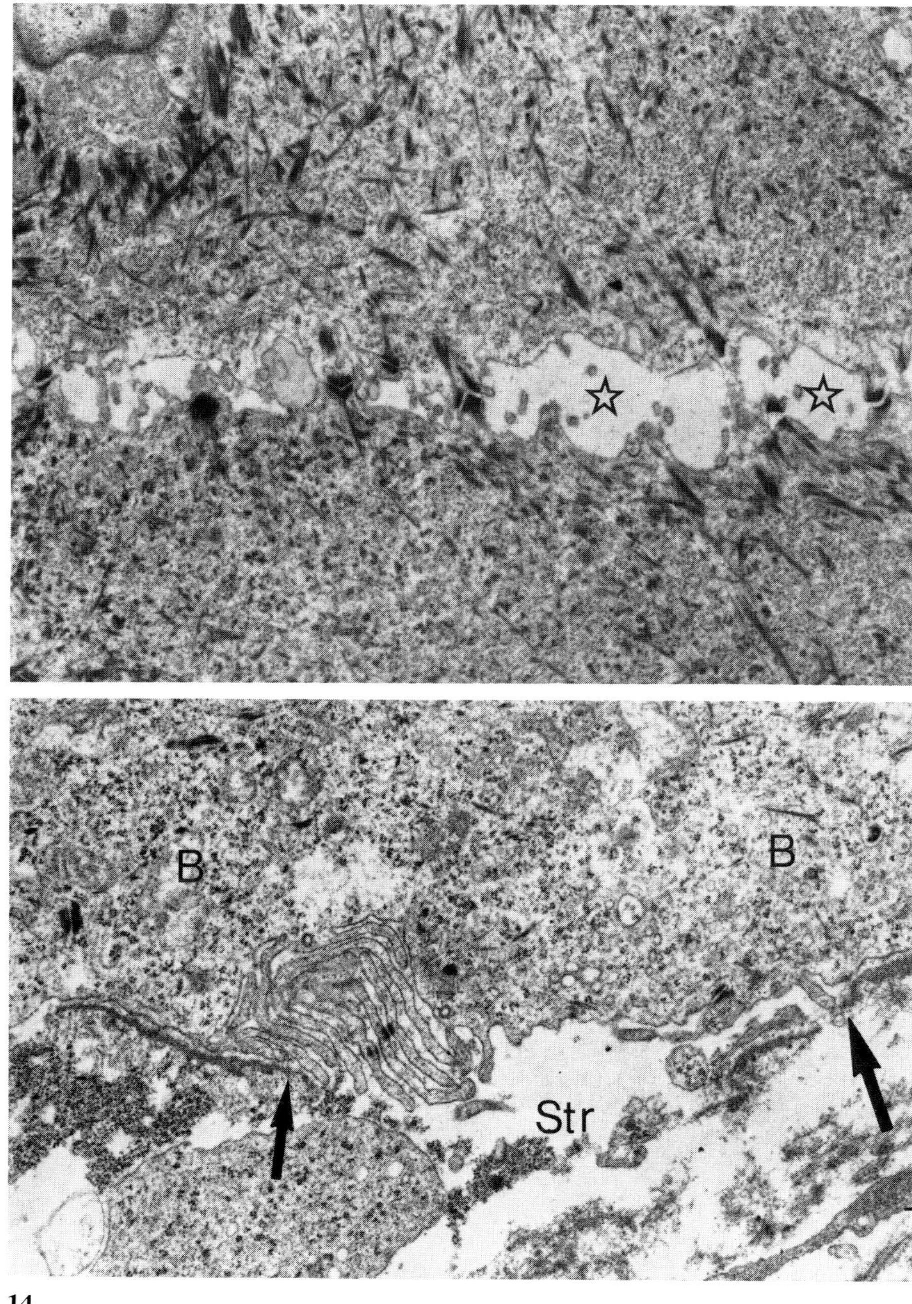

14

14 (top) Part of prickle cell layer, showing irregular alignment of tonofibrils and a marked reduction in desmosomal connections leading to development of intercellular spaces *(stars)*. (×9,100)

14 (below) Epithelial–mesenchymal interface (B = basal cells, Str = stroma) with basement membrane showing an extensive defect *(between arrows)*. The basement membrane is plicated in this region, indicating enhanced cell mobility. The phenomenon may be regarded as an ultrastructural microinvasion. (×14,000)

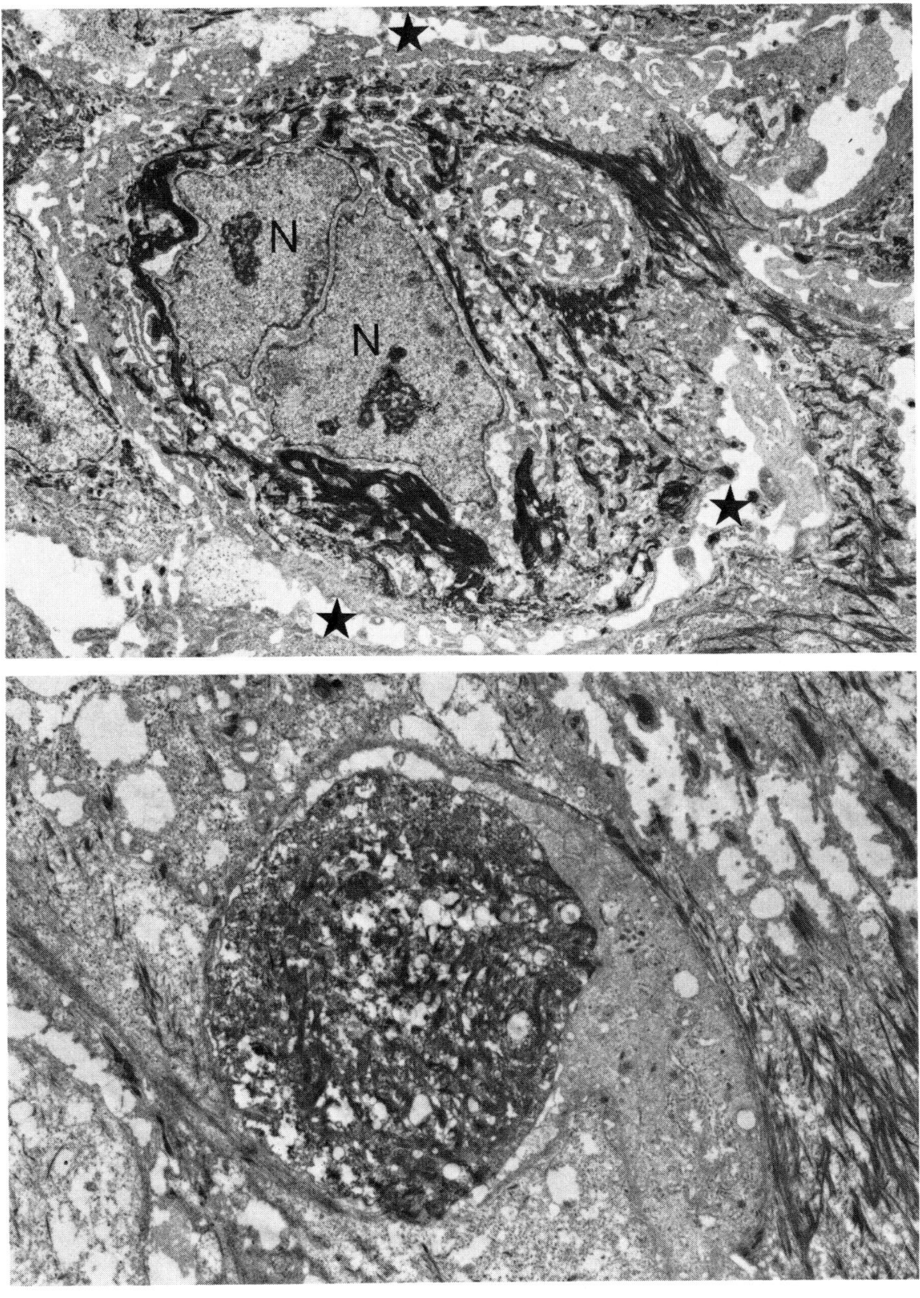

15

15 (top) Prickle cells with nuclei showing irregular lobulation, and two nucleoli (N). Cytoplasm contains thick, mainly perinuclear tonofibril bundles. Reduction in desmosomes and formation of intercellular spaces *(stars)* are evident. (×4,100)

15 (below) Dyskeratosis of spinous layer. Body of cell is rounded, the nucleus dissolved; cytoplasm contains dense aggregates of tonofibrils and remnants of cell organelles (dyskeratotic necrosis). (×4,900)

b) Leukoplakias with a moderate degree of dysplasia

These hold an intermediate position, having more marked dysplastic criteria (Table 7), and representing 17 per cent of leukoplakias. Their behaviour corresponds largely to that of the group with low-degree dysplasia, but the fact that there is more dysplasia should be taken into account when planning treatment.

Table 7 Grading of Dysplasia Criteria for a Classification According to Degree of Dysplasia, and Characteristics of Carcinoma *in situ*

Degree	Characteristics
Low	Basal cell hyperplasia Basal cell polarity disrupted
Medium	Basal cell hyperplasia Loss of basal cell polarity Moderate degree of pleomorphism Slight increase in rate of mitosis Occasional dyskeratosis
High	Basal cell hyperplasia Basal cell polarity lost Marked cellular pleomorphism Increase in rate of mitosis Numerous dyskeratoses Abnormal stratification of epithelium
Carcinoma *in situ*	Characteristics of high-degree dysplasia more marked Epithelial stratification lost Stroma not yet invaded

c) Leukoplakias with a high degree of dysplasia and carcinoma *in situ*

Leukoplakias with a high degree of dysplasia must be considered precancerous. They are identified by the fact that all the criteria of dysplasia are usually present in marked degree (Table 7). Endophytic growth with downward extension of epithelial rete pegs is a common finding.

Carcinoma *in situ* is characterised by the additional feature of complete loss of epithelial stratification. It may be regarded as an early form of oral cancer not showing invasive growth. Six per cent of leukoplakias show the signs of extreme dysplasia, three per cent those of carcinoma *in situ*.

Clinical experience has shown that about 10 per cent of leukoplakias are subject to malignant degeneration. The selected patient populations of specialist hospitals will, of course, show a higher incidence of dysplastic lesions (Table 8).

Table 8 Frequency of Different Degrees of Dysplasia in the Total Biopsy Material and in Selected Biopsy Material from an Oral Surgery Unit over a Period of Ten Years (%)

Degree of dysplasia	Total population (n = 656)	Oral surgery unit (n = 282)
No/low-degree dysplasia	74	63
Medium-degree dysplasia	17	17
Marked degree of dysplasia	6	16
Carcinoma *in situ*	3	4

d) 'Candida leukoplakia'

A secondary *Candida* infection of the epithelium may be found in about 10 per cent of all leukoplakias. If the degree of dysplasia is also taken into account, the incidence of candidiasis increases with the degree of dysplasia, reaching 38 per cent in lesions showing a high degree of dysplasia. Fungal growth in leukoplakic lesions must therefore be regarded both as a risk-factor and as a risk-indicator. Histologically, it is demonstrable by staining with periodic acid–Schiff (PAS) reagent. Apart from such invasion of the epithelium, *Candida albicans* occurs with even greater frequency quite generally in the oral cavity of leukoplakia patients. Mycological studies have demonstrated its presence in about half of such patients. In healthy control populations, the fungus is demonstrable in only half that number.

Clinical significance of the dysplasia classification – prognosis and treatment

The degree of dysplasia correlates with a number of clinical parameters that are known to relate to relatively poor prognosis. Such parameters are sex and age distribution, localisation, macroscopic appearance, the size of the lesion, the time for which it has persisted, the dental status, exogenous irritants and coincidence with oral carcinomata of different localisation. Figures **16** to **18** demonstrate the relationship between dysplasia classification and prognosis. Only three per cent of patients with mucosal lesions showing no, or only a minor degree of dysplasia, and four per cent of patients with a moderate degree of dysplasia developed malignancies. Whereas, 43 per cent of patients showing a high degree of epithelial dysplasia and carcinoma *in situ* developed oral carcinoma. Even after total removal of all mucosal tissue showing macroscopic changes, leukoplakia with dysplasia must be regarded as indicating a tendency to dysplasia and malignant degeneration that may affect other areas of the mucosa. Recurrences and the development of cancer have been noted under these circumstances (multifocal or multicentric carcinogenesis). Close and effective follow-up care is therefore necessary for leukoplakia with marked dysplasia, even following radical removal of the lesions.

— *Continued on page 80*

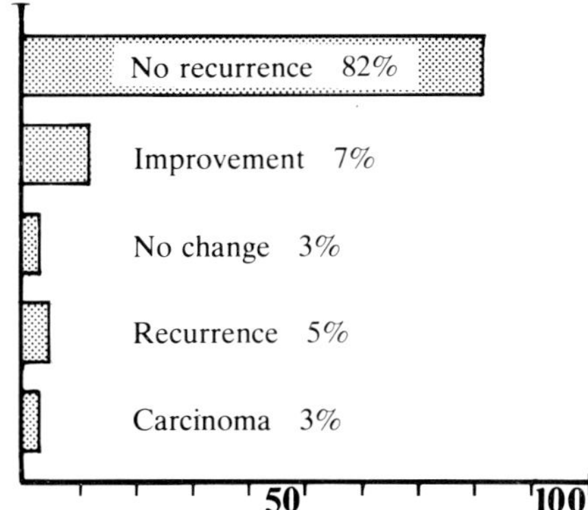

16 Clinical progress of patients with oral leukoplakia involving no, or only a minor degree of dysplasia (n = 129).

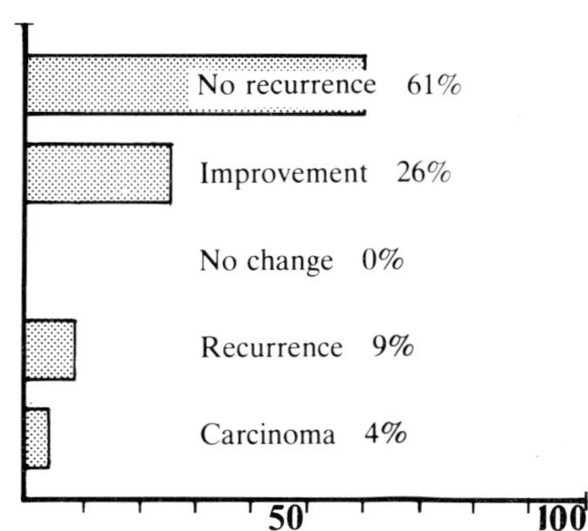

17 Clinical progress of patients with oral leukoplakia showing a moderate degree of dysplasia (n = 31).

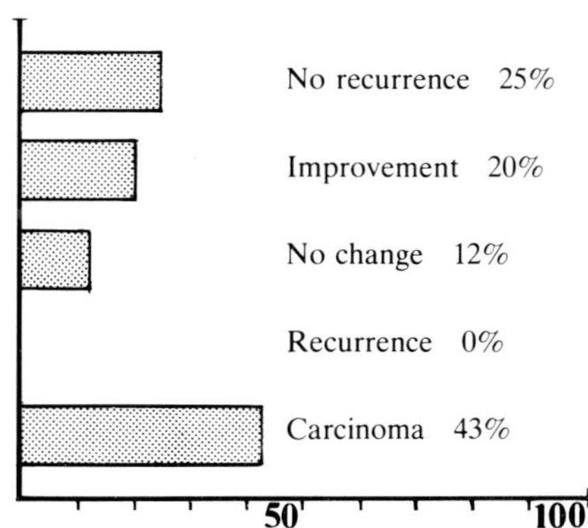

18 Clinical progress of patients with oral leukoplakia showing a high degree of dysplasia (including carcinoma *in situ*; n = 40).

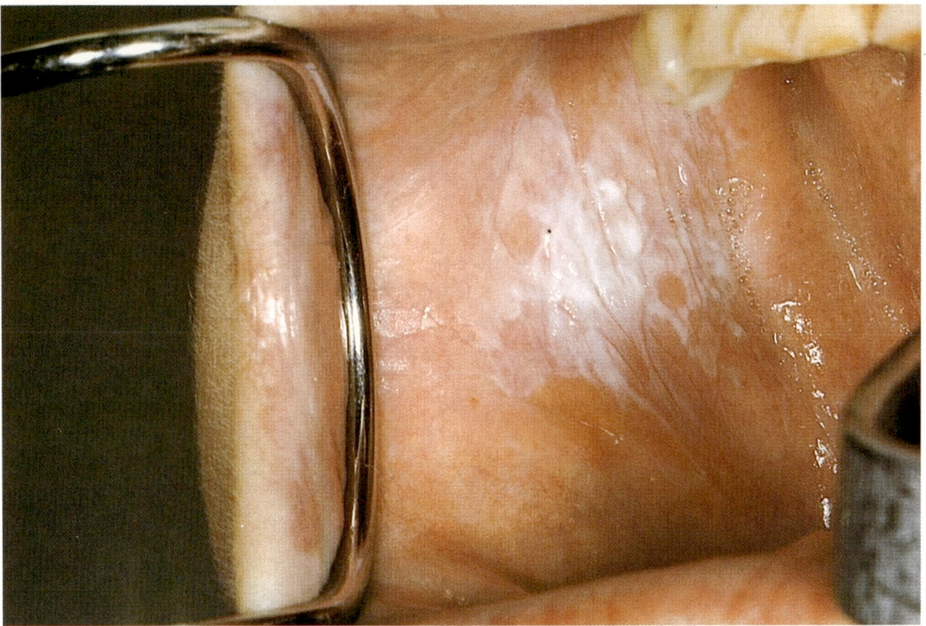

19

19 Homogeneous, whitish discoloration that cannot be rubbed off, in the buccal mucosa. Fine, non-hypertrophic extensions can be seen at the point of transition to normal mucosa. There is no infiltration or ulceration. (Female aged 58; clinically non-suspect)

20 Normally stratified planar epithelium with rete pegs slightly deeper than normal. Prickle cell layer is increased (acanthosis). Horny surface layer shows loosened structure. There is loose connective tissue and no cell proliferation.

21 Greater magnification shows a slight increase in basal cells. Above are prickle cells containing plenty of glycogen. *(PAS)*

22 Detail from horny layer showing considerable sponginess with fairly large pools of fluid between the horny lamellae ('keratin pools'). This type of change is seen particularly frequently with 'leukoedema'.

Clinical management

Exclusion of risk-factors, followed by conservative treatment and observation. Biopsy is not required where the lesion is completely harmless clinically, but will become necessary if there is progression. Follow-up observation should be undertaken in the course of general treatment procedures.

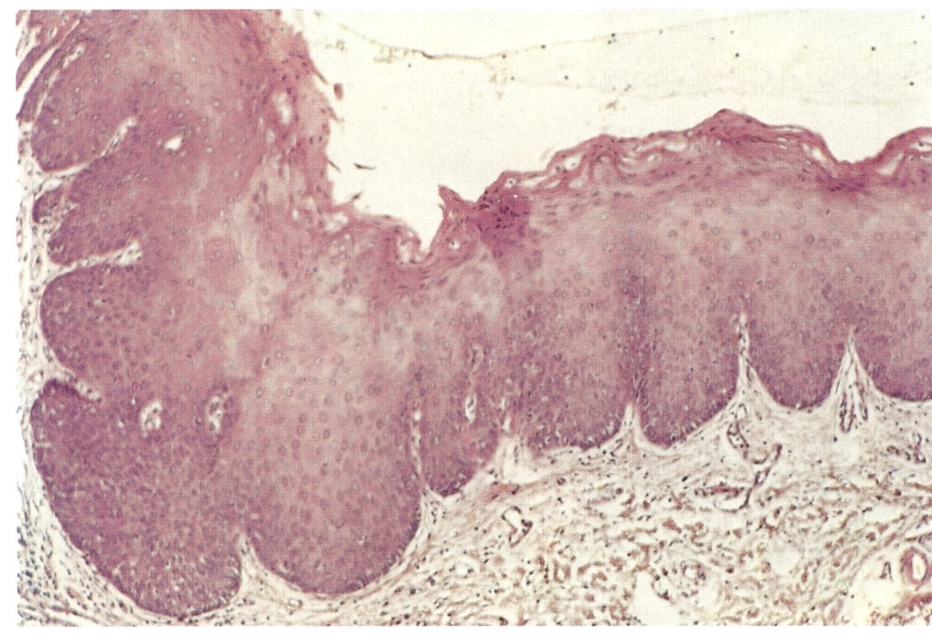

20

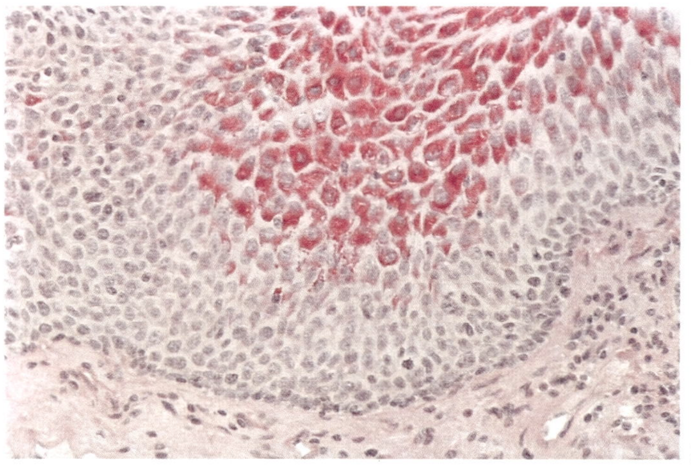

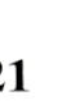

21

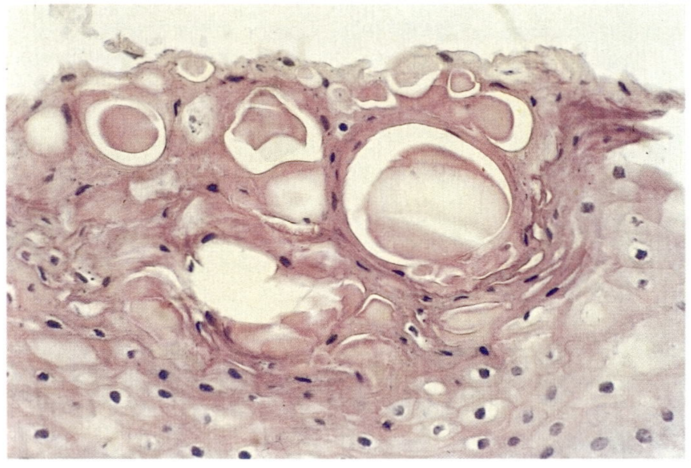

22

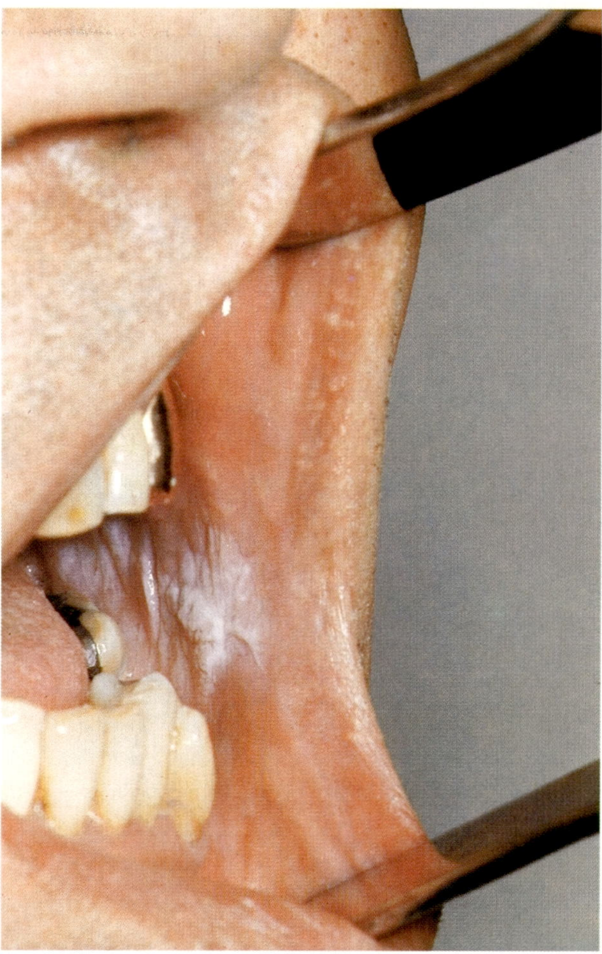

23

23 Somewhat more marked whitish discoloration, partly in the form of striations, that cannot be rubbed off, in the region of the intercalary line of the left buccal mucosa. Surface appearance is homogeneous. (Male aged 50; clinically non-suspect)

24 Planar epithelium, slightly increased, with regular stratification. There is a wide band of orthokeratosis (anucleate horny layer, stained an even red). Beneath lies a shallow granular layer. Connective tissue is loose and cell proliferation is not marked.

25 Normal basal cell layer, with polar arrangement. Prickle cell layer is normal. Loose connective tissue can be seen, with fine capillaries immediately beneath the epithelium.

26 Greater magnification shows normal basal cell layer and above it prickle cells with consistent rounded nuclei.

Clinical management

Exclusion of risk-factors, followed by conservative treatment and observation. Biopsy is not required where the lesion is completely harmless clinically, but will become necessary if there is progression. Follow-up observation should be undertaken in the course of general treatment procedures.

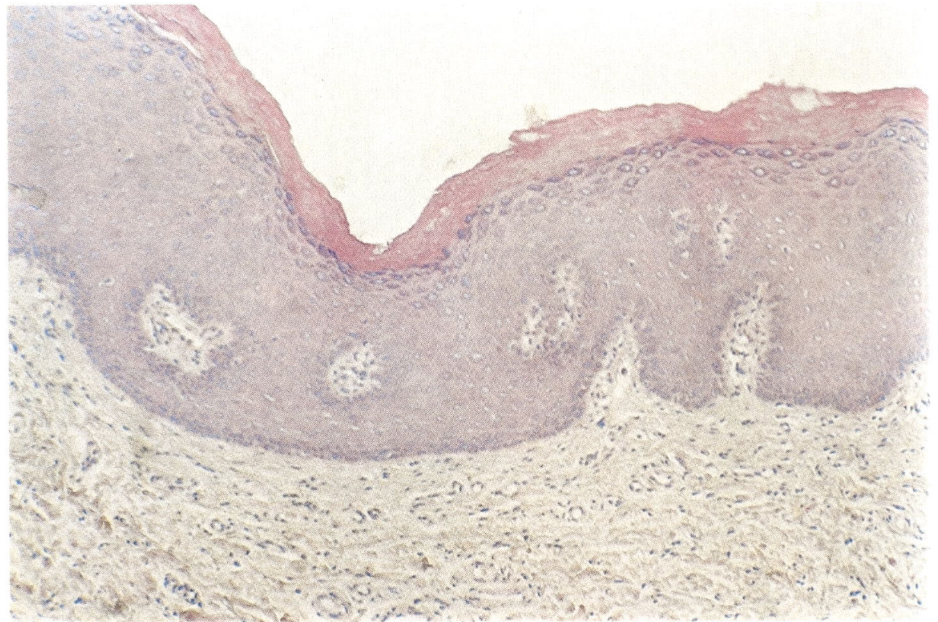

24

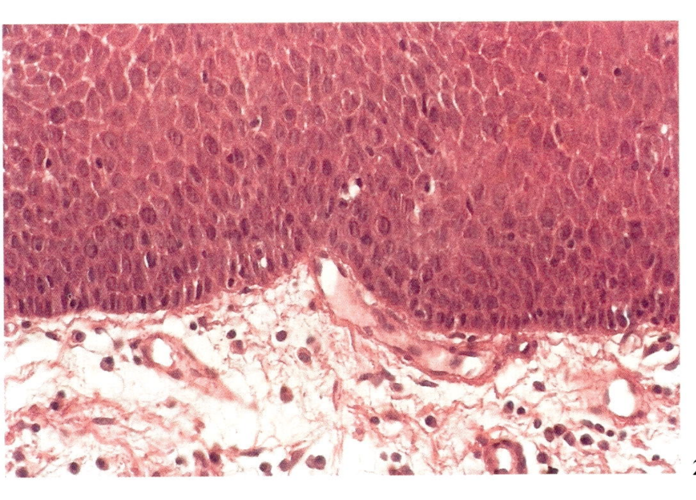

25

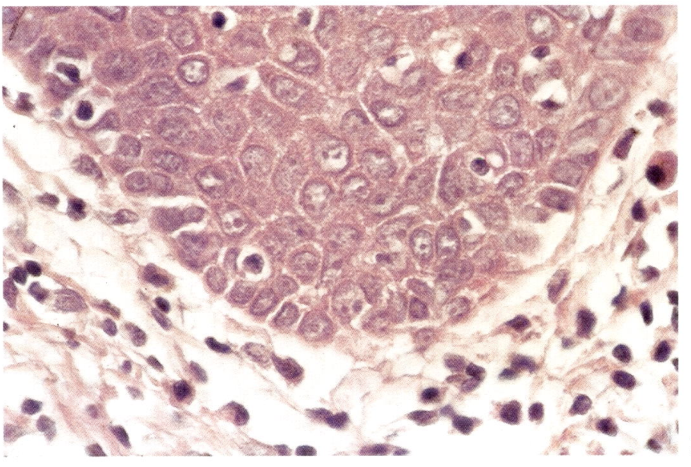

26

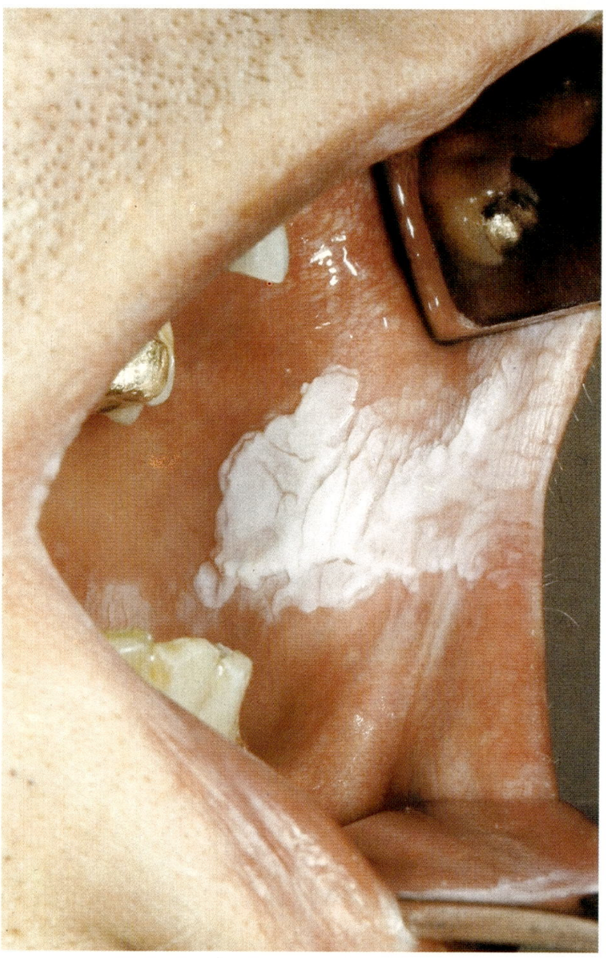

27

27 Sharply circumscribed, thickened whitish lesion in the mucosa, retroangular and extending into the buccal plane. Lesion does not rub off; surface appearance is homogeneous and broken up by small longitudinal fissures. There is no infiltration or ulceration. (Male aged 61; clinically non-suspect)

28 Planar epithelium showing regular stratification, with a slight increase in rete peg formation. Prickle cell layer is slightly increased (acanthosis). Superficially there is a wide parakeratotic horny layer with remnants of nuclei still discernible. Loose connectve tissue can be seen subepithelially.

29 Detail showing marked increase in basal cell population, with a normal prickle cell layer. Subepithelial connective tissue is stained green. *(Masson–Goldner)*

30 Epithelial rete with irregular basal cell hyperplasia and polar arrangement lost in parts. Subepithelial connective tissue in this region shows slight increase in round cell infiltration.

Clinical management

In view of the extent and degree of the lesion, regression is unlikely. Excision, at least in part, is necessary, as is determination of the degree of dysplasia. In the case in Figures **27** to **30**, dysplasia is minimal. After exclusion of risk-factors (no smoking, better oral hygiene) and conservative treatment of the residual lesion, follow-up at reasonable intervals will be sufficient.

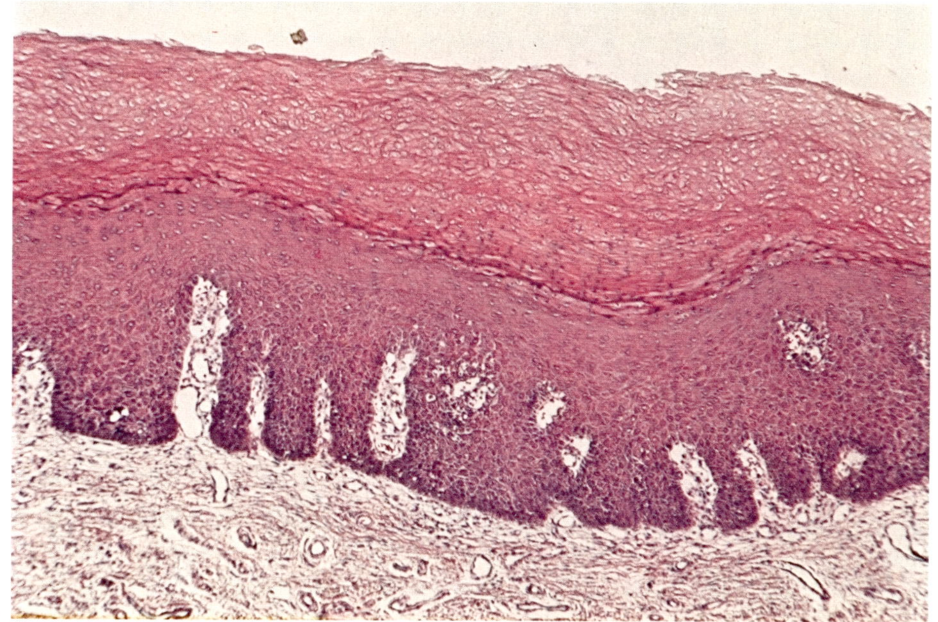
28

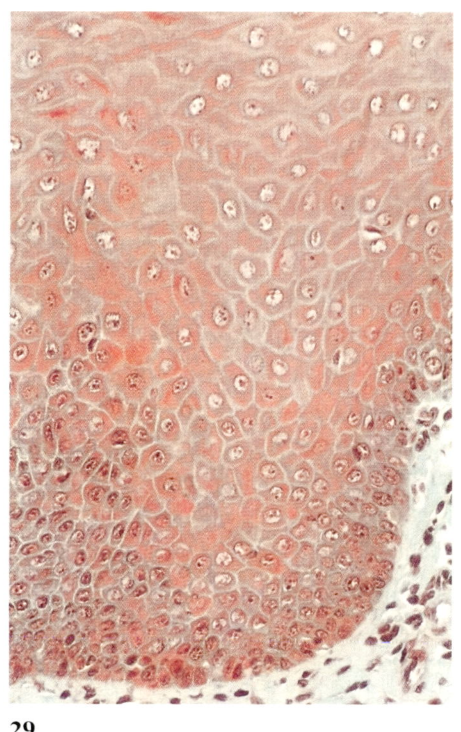
29

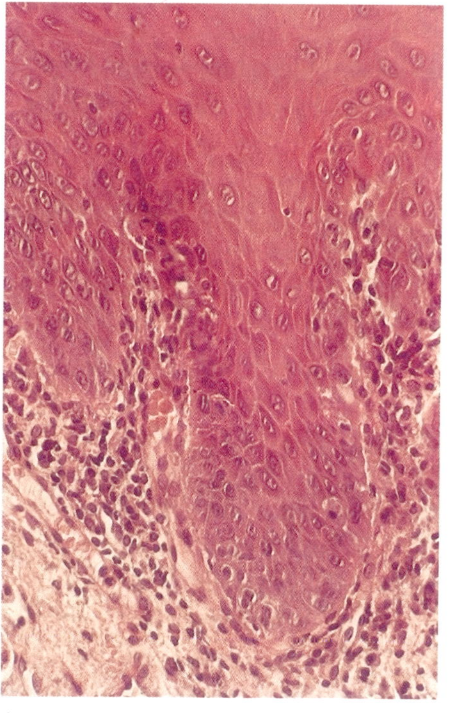
30

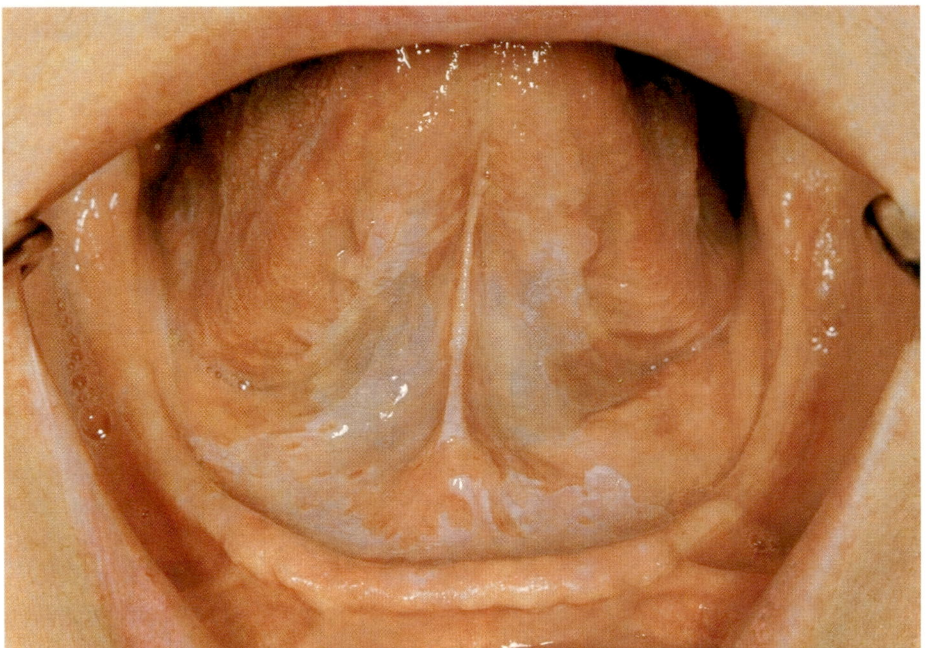

31

31 Extremely fine, non-hypertrophic, homogeneous whitish discoloration on the underside of the tongue and mucosa of the floor of the mouth, feathering in the margins. There is no ulceration or infiltration. (Female aged 66; clinically non-suspect)

32 Planar epithelium with normal stratification and basal limit sharply defined. There is slight basal cell hyperplasia and a moderate degree of acanthosis, with a loose-structured parakeratotic horny layer.

33 PAS staining reveals abundant intracellular glycogen. Only the basal cell layer is free from glycogen. Such an abundance of glycogen largely excludes any marked degree of epithelial dysplasia. *(PAS)*

34 Greater magnification shows basal cell proliferation and, superficial to this, oedematous (ballooning) prickle cells. These changes represent nonspecific epithelial damage.

Clinical management

Exclusion of risk-factors, followed by conservative treatment and observation. Biopsy is not required where the lesion is completely harmless clinically, but will become necessary if there is progression. Follow-up obervation should be undertaken in the course of general treatment procedures.

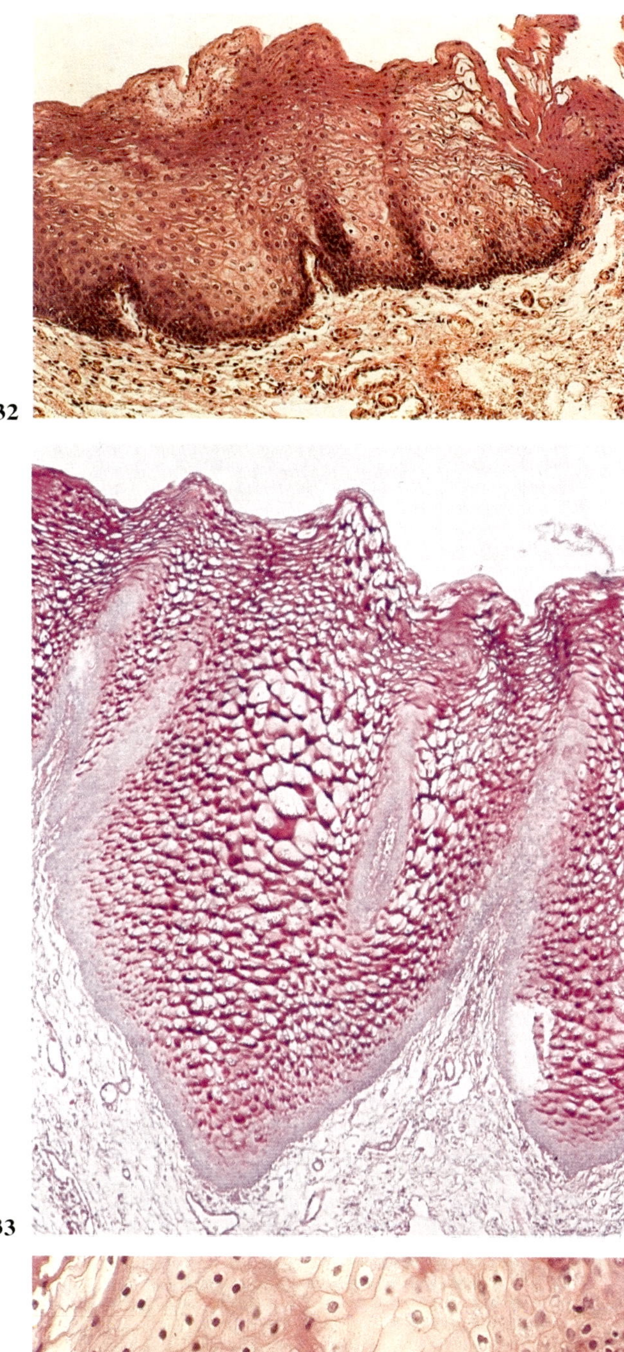

32

33

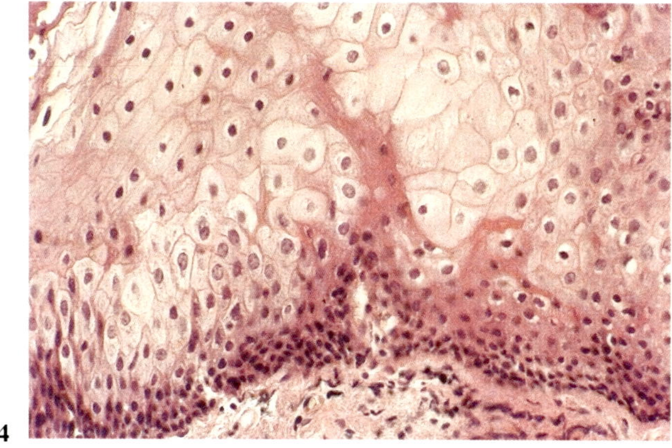

34

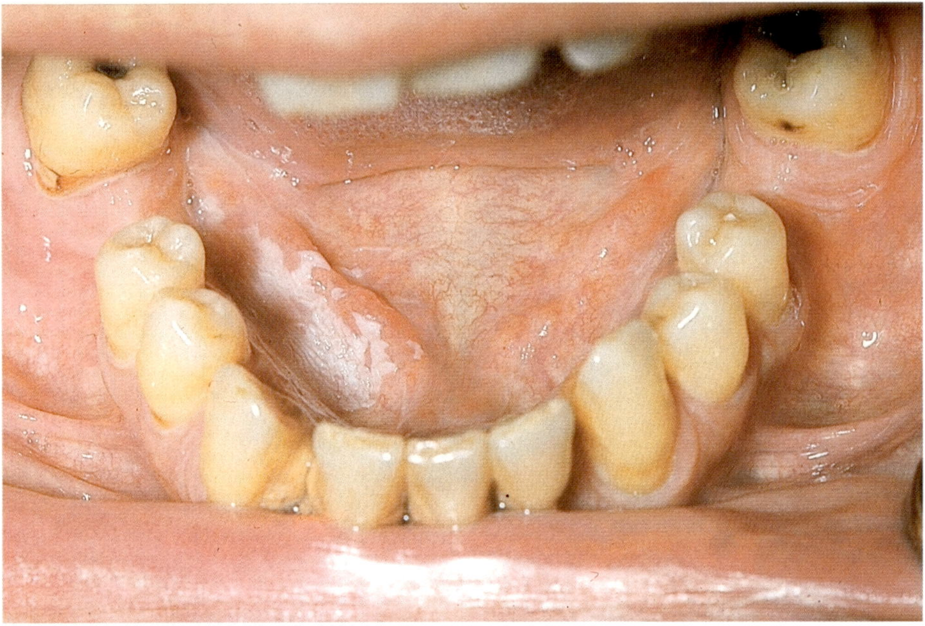

35

35 Very white homogeneous discoloration of mucosa on floor of the mouth, on the right in the region of sublingual fold, with no ulceration or infiltration. (Male aged 42; clinically non-suspect)

36 Planar epithelium showing normal stratification, with acanthosis and extensive orthokeratosis. Granular cell layer is clearly visible. Superficially, the horny layer is thick, with only occasional shadow nuclei. Subepithelially, there is a slight increase in round cells.

37 Surface mucosa at greater magnification, showing granular cell layer with clearly discernible granules. Horny layer is loose-structured and largely anucleate.

38 Light-microscopic basement membrane demonstrated by silvering. Beneath the polar arrangement of basal cells lies a clearly visible meshwork of fibres.

Clinical management

Exclusion of risk-factors, followed by conservative treatment and observation. Biopsy is not required where the lesion is completely harmless clinically, but will become necessary if there is progression. Follow-up observation should be undertaken in the course of general treatment procedures.

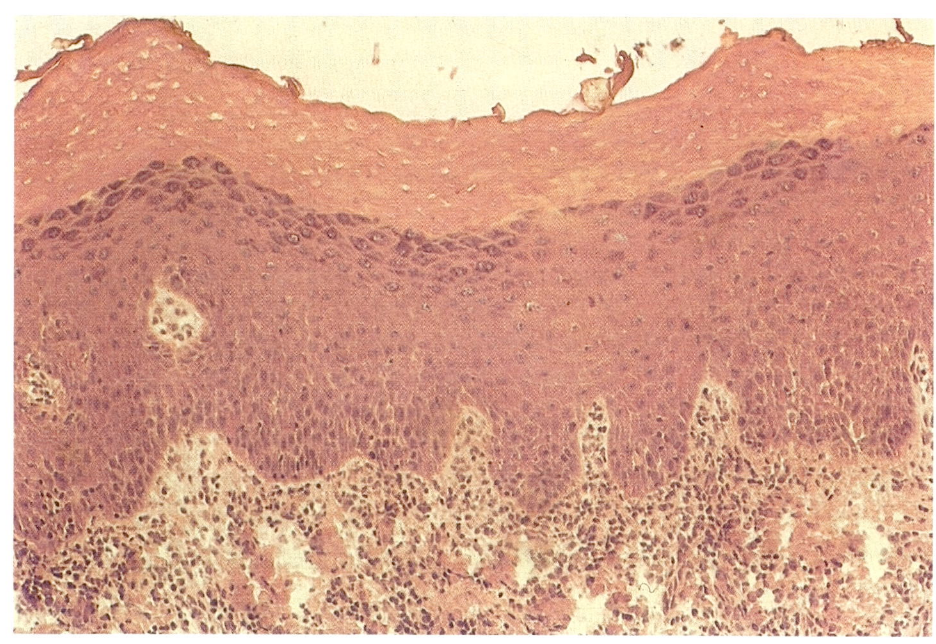

36

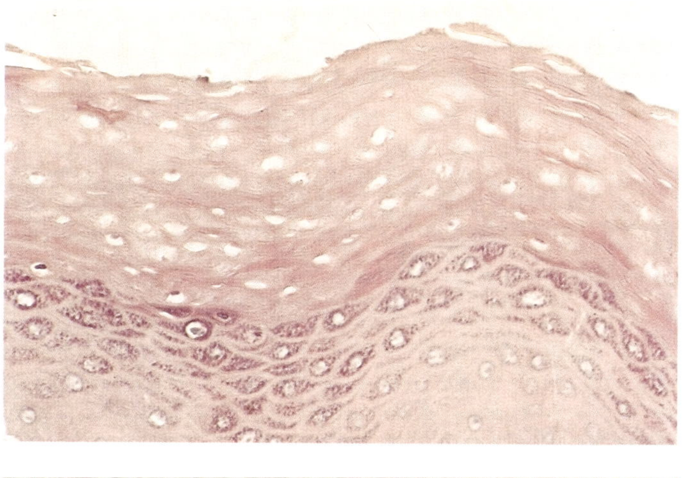

37

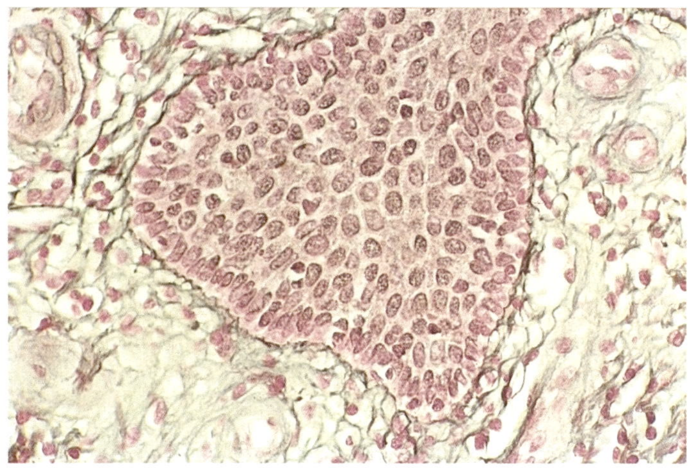

38

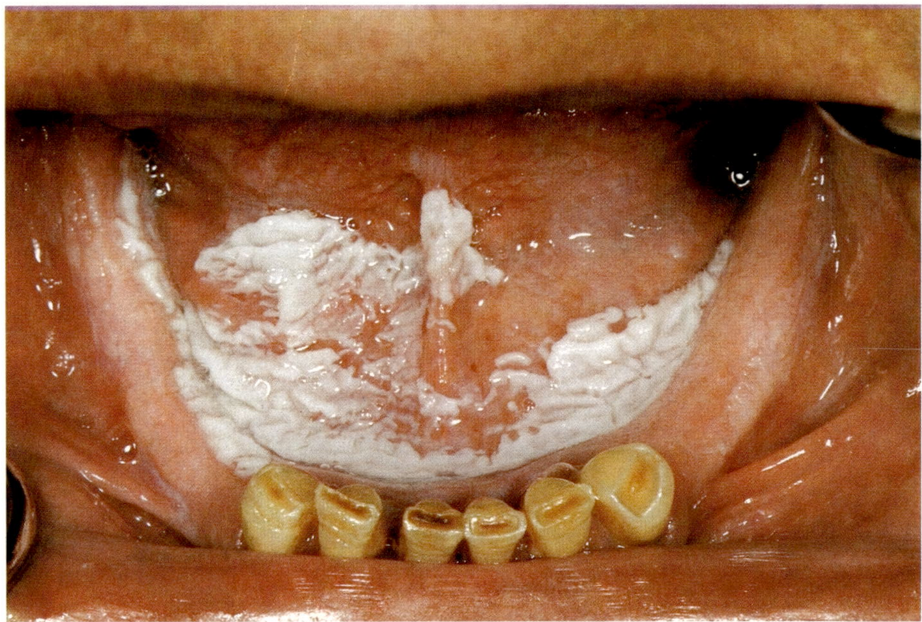

39

39 Thick whitish change, its surface homogeneous, involving mucosa of the whole floor of the mouth and lingual surface of the alveolar process in the lower jaw. There is a wave-like variation in the surface (ebb-tide leukoplakia). (Female aged 58; clinically non-suspect)

40 Greatly thickened planar epithelium with normal stratification and a wide zone of hyperorthokeratosis showing focal enhancement. Low-degree fibrosis is present subepithelially.

41 Downward extension of rete pegs, anastomosing in parts. Broad granular and horny layers are clearly visible.

42 Greater magnification shows focal loss of polar arrangement of basal cells. Suprabasally there is a mitotic figure.

Clinical management

In view of the extent and severity of the lesion, regression is unlikely. This, and the risk-factor of localisation in the floor of the mouth, necessitate excision, at least in part, and determination of the degree of dysplasia. After exclusion of risk-factors (no smoking, better oral hygiene) and conservative treatment of the residual lesion, follow-up at reasonable intervals will be sufficient.

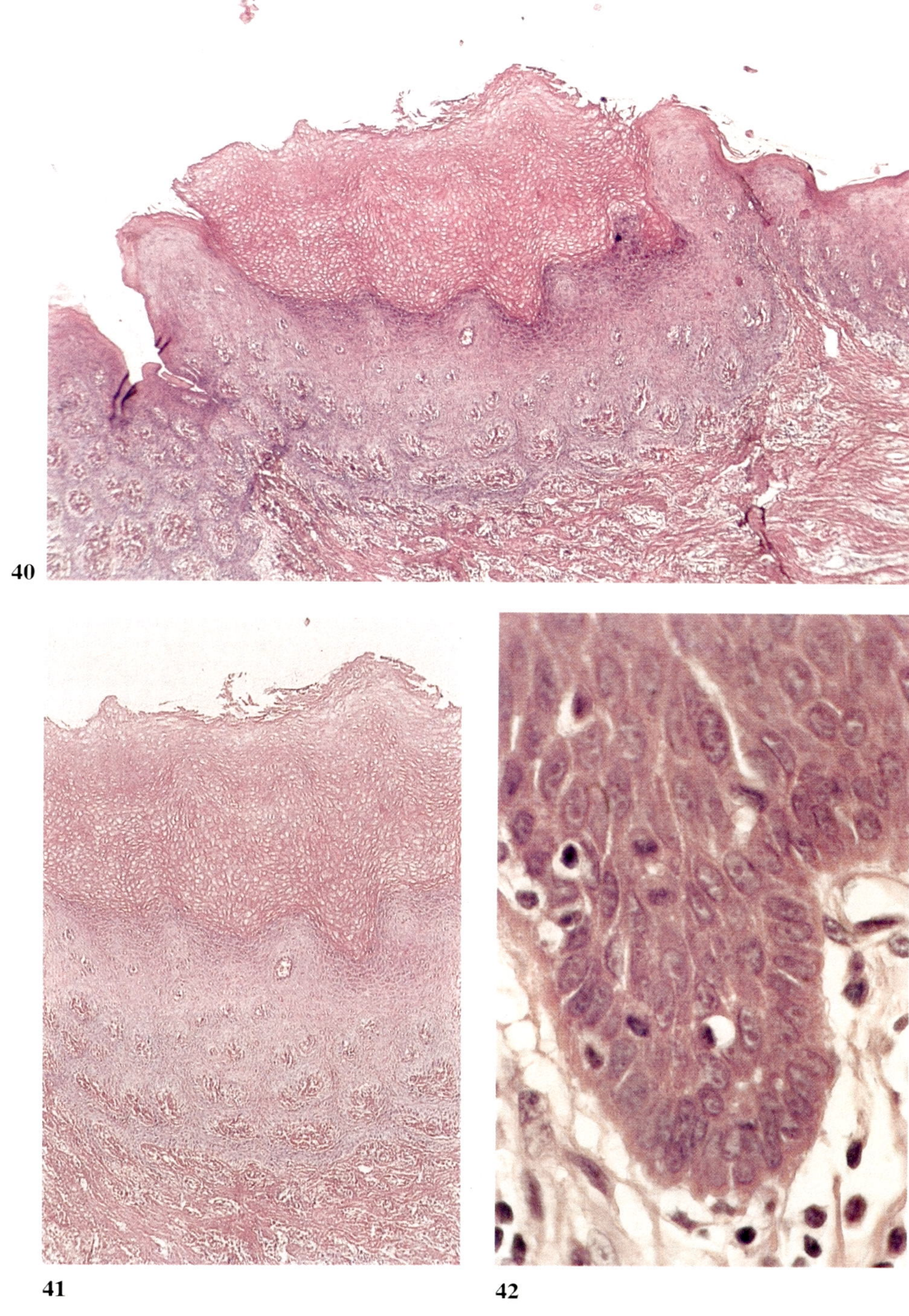

40

41

42

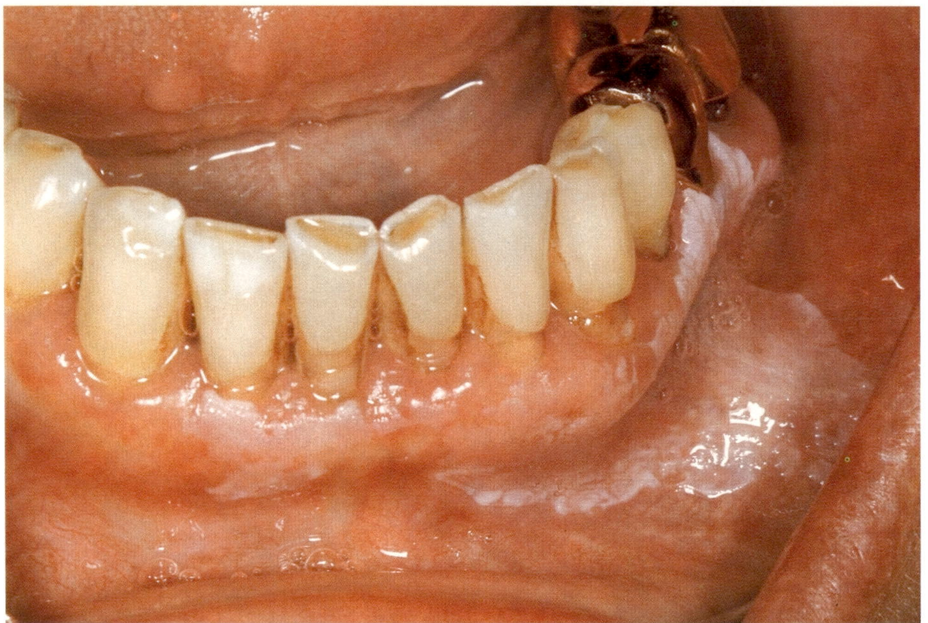

43

43 Fine, whitish change in the mucosa in the region of the attached gingiva and part of the free gingiva of the mandibular vestibule, with no infiltration or ulceration. (Female aged 67; clinically non-suspect)

44 Planar epithelium with normal stratification and low-grade focal basal cell hyperplasia. At the surface there is a change from hyperorthokeratosis (left) to hyperparakeratosis (right).

45 Basal part of epithelium showing normal structure.

46 Greater magnification shows well established polar arrangement of basal cells. Prickle cells are normal in appearance, and nuclei are regular in size, taking normal stain. Subepithelially, occasional round cells are in evidence.

Clinical management

Exclusion of risk-factors, followed by conservative treatment and observation. Biopsy is not required where the lesion is completely harmless clinically, but will become necessary if there is progression. Follow-up observation should be undertaken in the course of general treatment procedures.

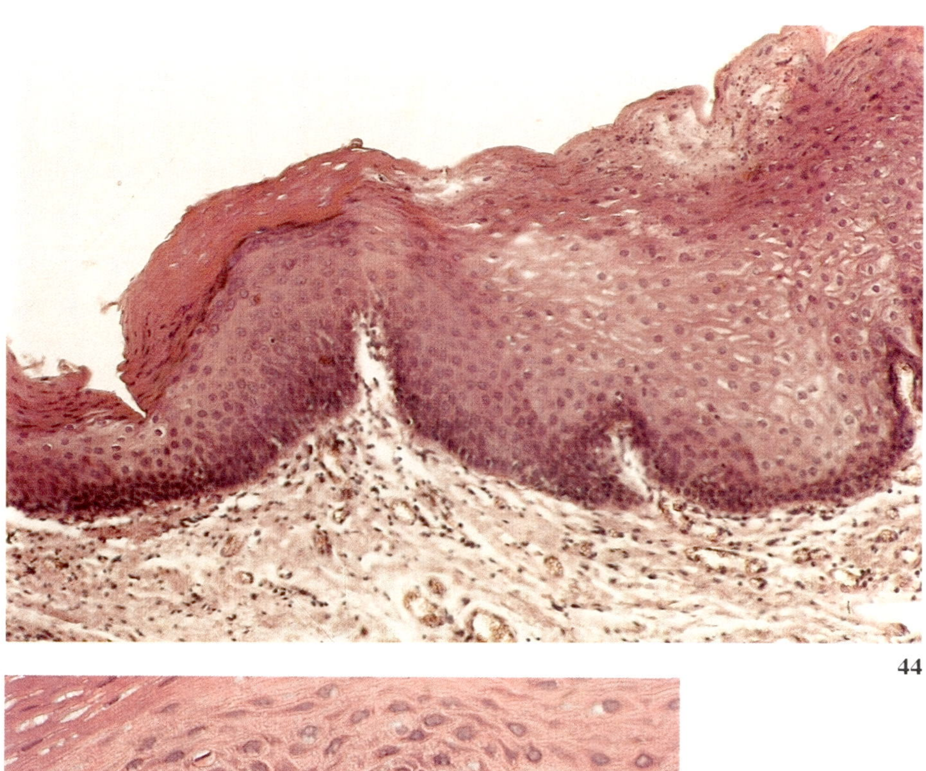

44

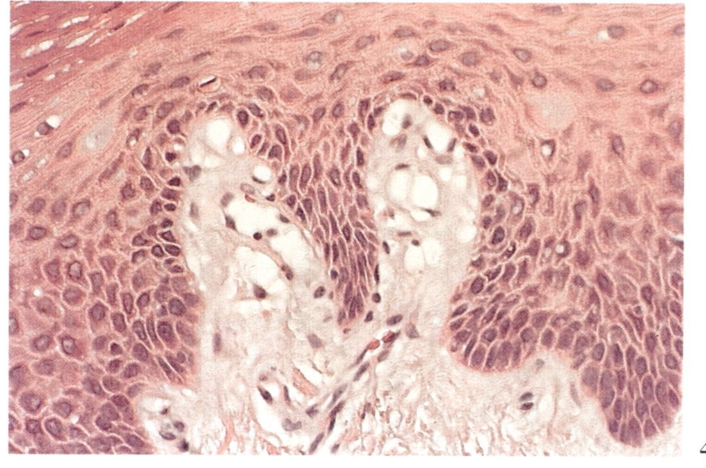

45

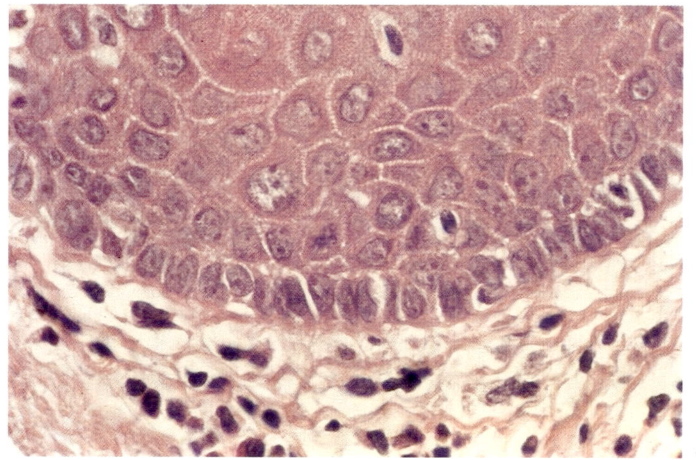

46

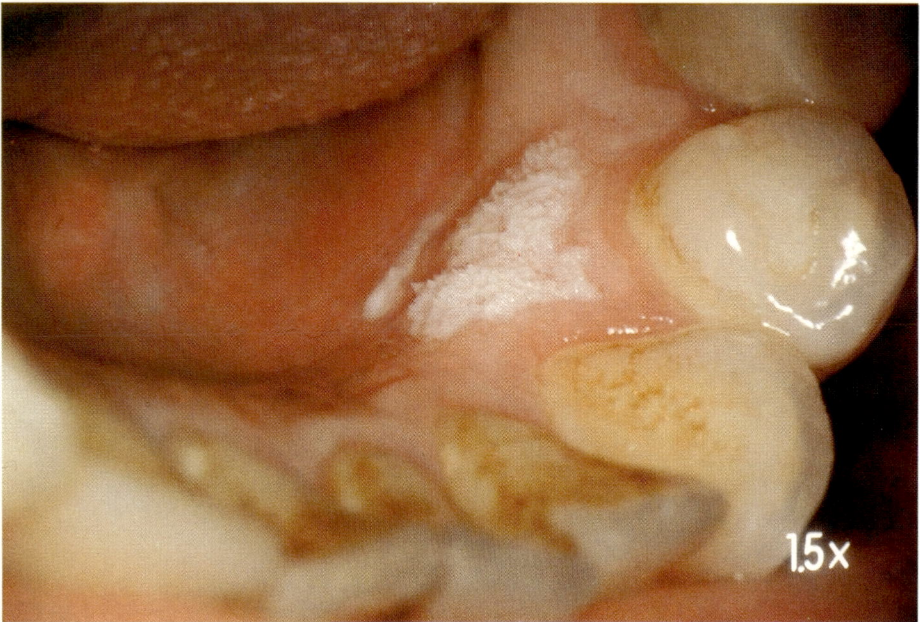

47

47 A sharply defined, slightly hypertrophic whitish change in the mucosa, with granular surface structure, lingual to canine and first mandibular premolar in the region of the attached gum. There is no infiltration or ulceration. (Female aged 24; clinically non-suspect)

48 Papillomatous exophytic epithelium showing normal stratification of epithelium. There is a broad band of hyperorthokeratosis, with shadow nuclei persisting in part. Increased inflammatory infiltration has occurred subepithelially.

49 Saw-toothed papillary epithelial configuration clearly in evidence.

50 Basal portion of a rete peg showing normal basal cells but slightly loosened structure. Immediately inferior to this are round cell infiltrates which, in the area of the tip of the rete peg, also extend into the epithelium.

Clinical management

Exclusion of risk-factors, followed by conservative treatment and observation. Biopsy is not required where the lesion is completely harmless clinically, but will become necessary if there is progression. Follow-up observation should be undertaken in the course of general treatment procedures.

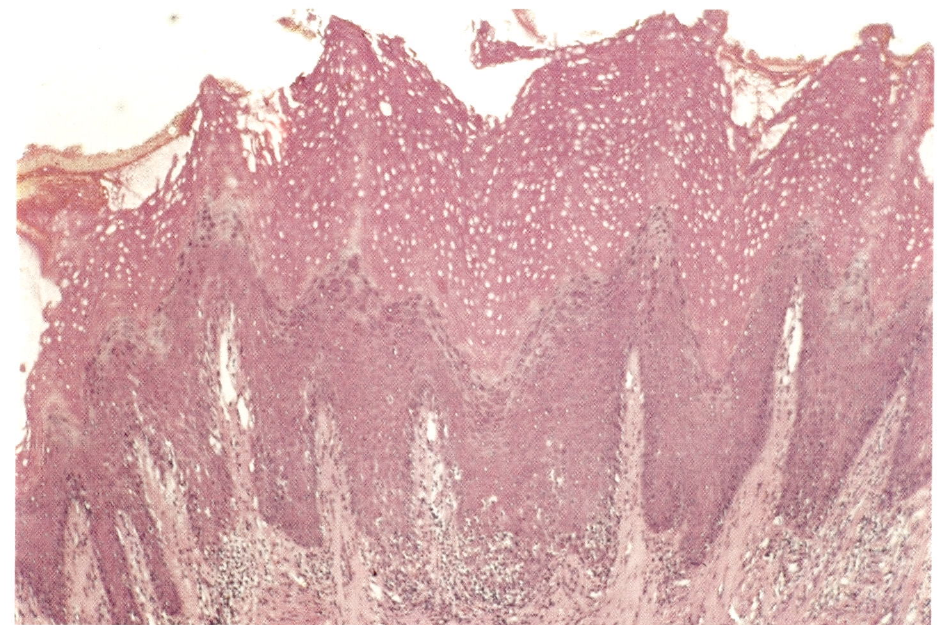
48

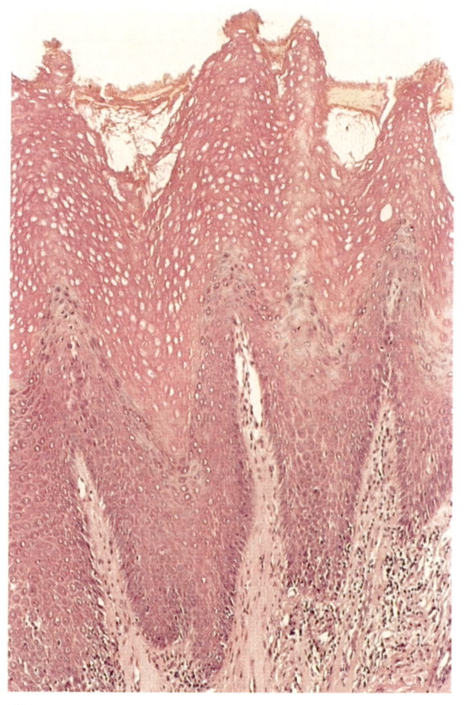
49

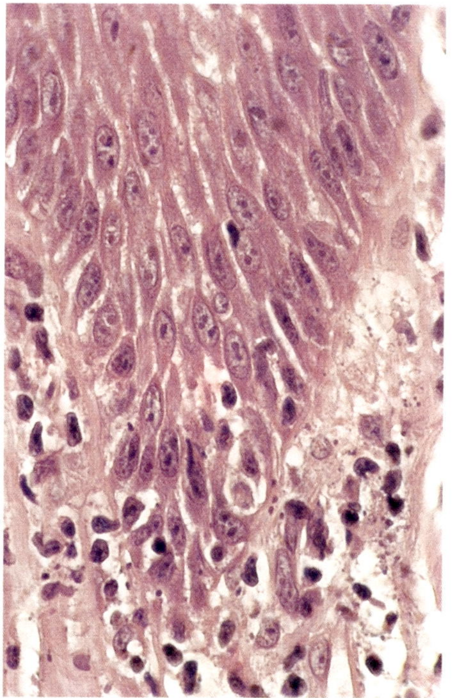
50

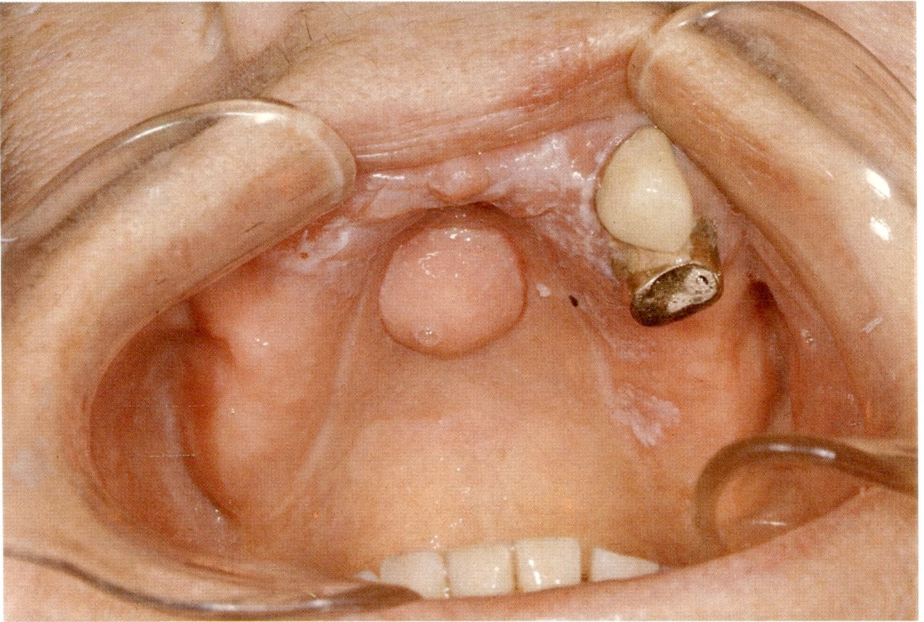

51

51 Diffuse whitish discoloration, that cannot be rubbed off, in the region of the alveolar ridge of the maxilla and of the palatal mucosa, beneath a partial upper denture. The lesion is concurrent with pedunculate fibroma in the denture margin in the central palate. (Male aged 63; clinically non-suspect)

52 Planar epithelium with normal stratification, polar basal cells, a slight increase in prickle cell layer and hyperparakeratosis. Stratum granulosum is not discernible. Low-degree fibrosis of subepithelial connective tissue is evident.

53 High-power micrograph of shallow rete pegs showing only occasional loss of polarity in basal cells.

54 Light-microscopic basement membrane, well represented as a broad band stained red immediately adjacent to basal cells. *(PAS)*

Clinical management

Exclusion of risk-factors followed by conservative treatment. As the condition is entirely harmless clinically, there is no need for a biopsy, though it will be required if there is progression. Fibroma should be excised and new dentures fitted. Follow-up observation should be undertaken as part of general treatment programme.

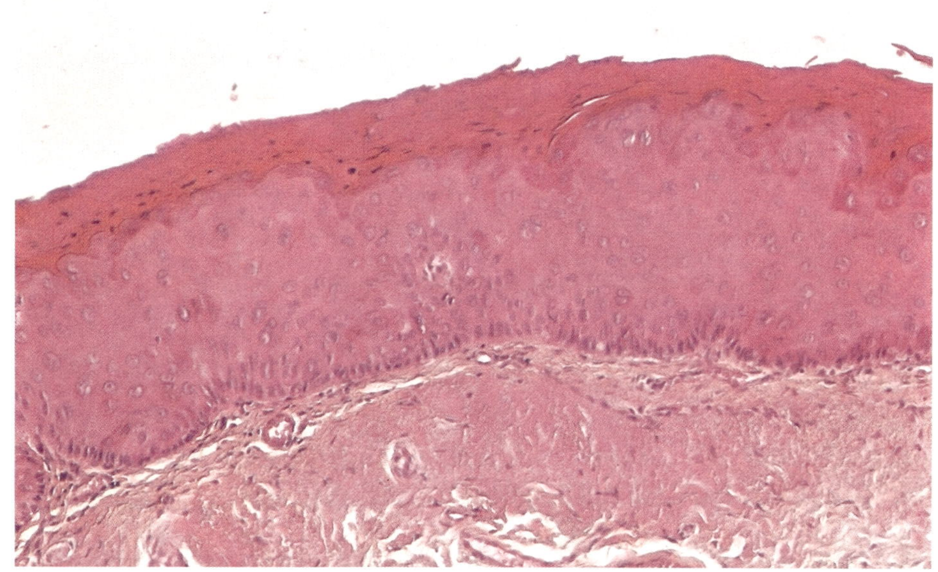
52

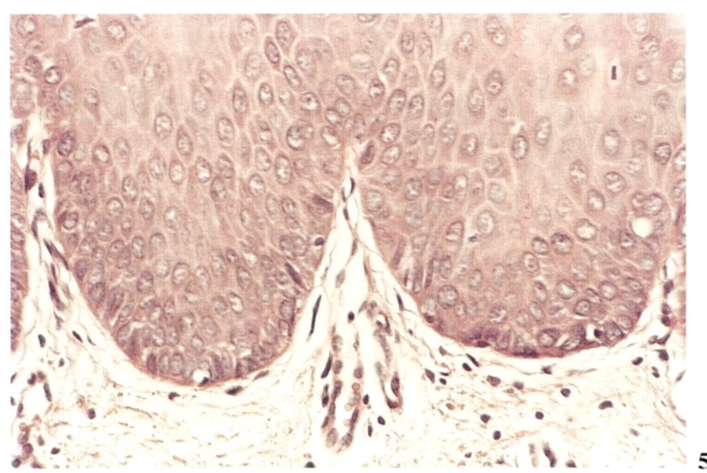
53

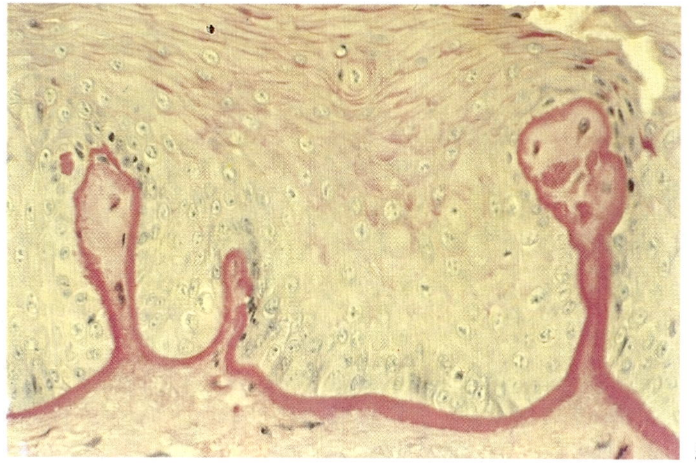
54

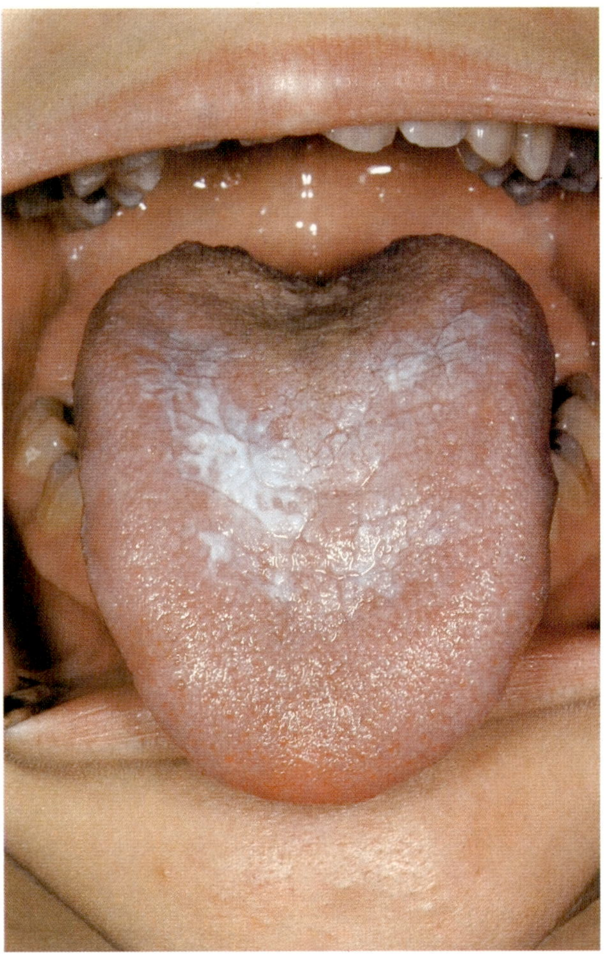

55

55 Homogeneous whitish discoloration of the dorsum of the tongue that cannot be rubbed off, with diffuse and indistinct margins and enhanced surface relief structure. (Female aged 16, cigarette smoker; clinically non-suspect)

56 Papillomatous epithelium showing exophytic proliferation, with acanthosis and marked hyperparakeratosis.

57 Normal differentiation of epithelium in the region of the rete pegs, with a slight degree of subepithelial fibrosis. *(Masson–Goldner)*

58 Greater magnification shows only a slight increase in basal cell layer. Superior to this are fusiform prickle cells.

Clinical management

Exclusion of risk-factors, followed by conservative treatment and observation. Biopsy is not required where the lesion is completely harmless clinically, but will become necessary if there is progression. Follow-up observation should be undertaken in the course of general treatment procedures.

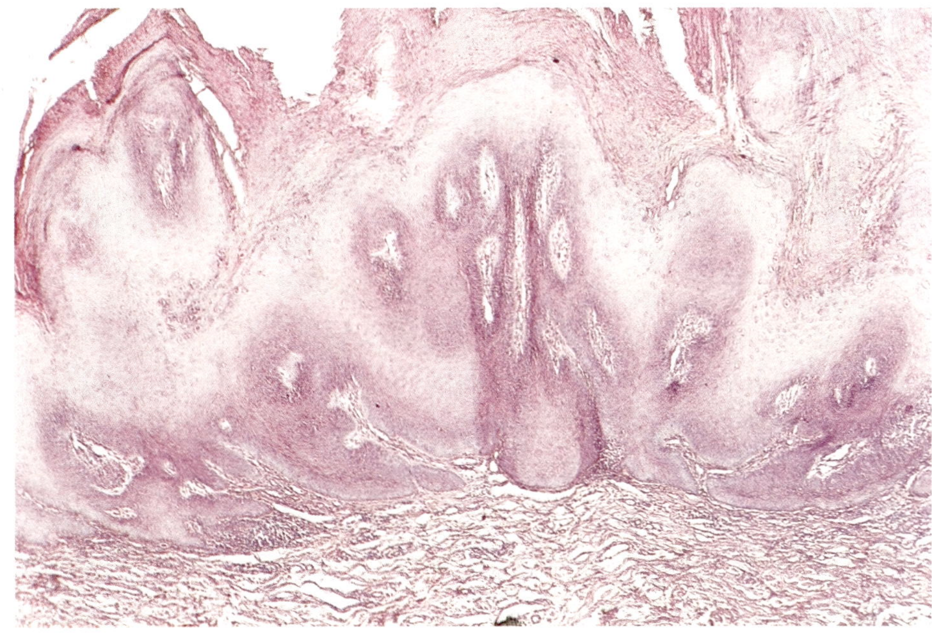

56

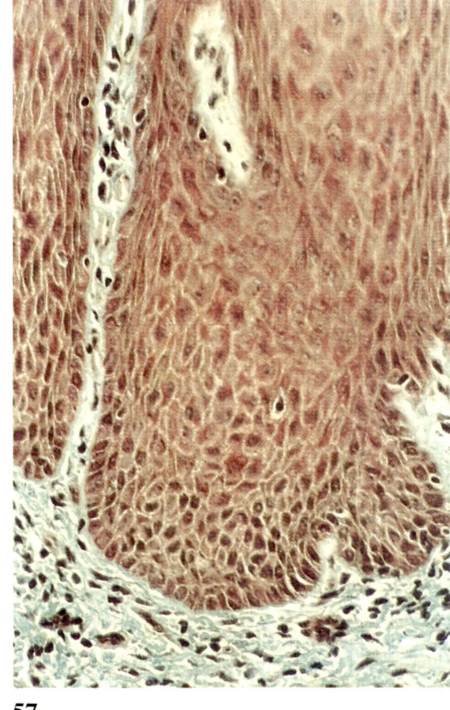

57

58

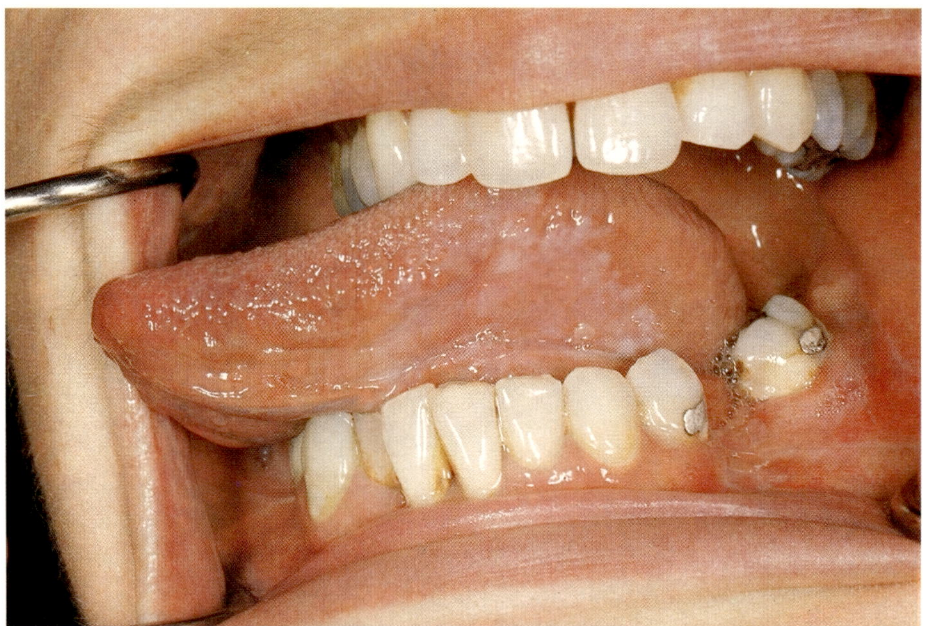

59

59 Homogeneous, faintly whitish discoloration of mucosa of the tongue, with no ulceration or infiltration. (Female aged 39; clinically non-suspect)

60 Planar epithelium showing some degree of convolution, with normal stratification and hyperorthokeratosis. Round cell infiltrates in connective tissue are slightly increased.

61 Shallow rete pegs with low-degree basal cell hyperplasia and marked acanthosis.

62 In this area, rete pegs are more developed and epithelial differentiation is maintained.

Clinical management

Exclusion of risk-factors followed by conservative treatment and observation. As the condition is clinically harmless, there is no need for a biopsy, providing the condition regresses. The tongue being a risk area, follow-up observation is indicated.

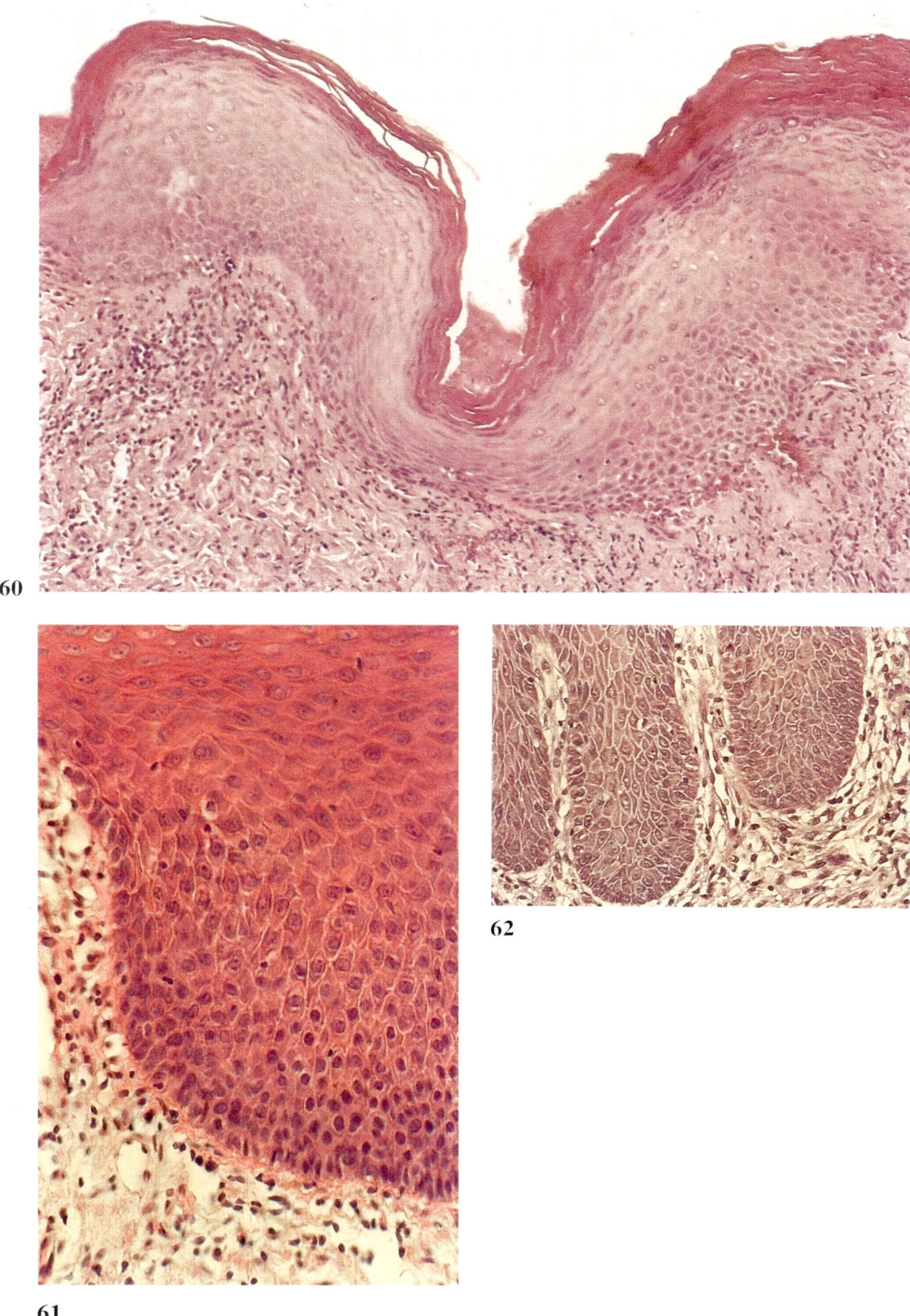

60

61

62

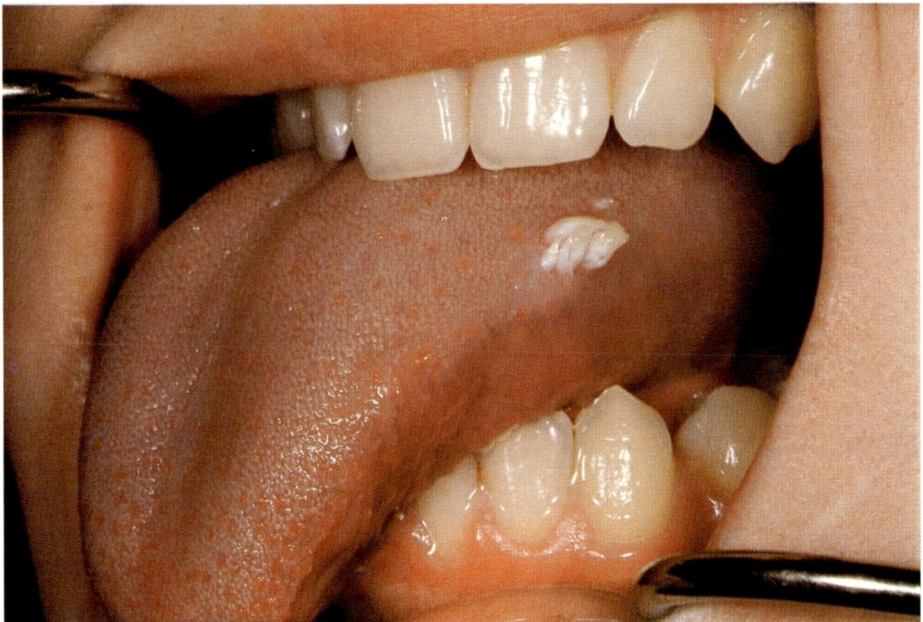

63

63 Homogeneous whitish discoloration, that cannot be rubbed off, in surface of mucosal papilloma. Mucosa is otherwise n.a.d. (Female aged 13; clinically non-suspect)

64 Normal epithelium with orthokeratosis (left) continuing into an area of extensive exophytic growth, with acanthosis and a broadened, very loosely structured parakeratotic horny layer.

65 Papillomatous projection of epithelium, with a narrow cone of connective tissue. There is a broad band of hyperkeratosis and the granular layer is not discernible.

66 Detail from the basal portion of the epithelium showing normal differentiation of basal cell layer. Basal cell hyperplasia is focal and of minor degree. Nuclei are regular and round, taking normal stain.

Clinical management

Excision of papilloma into healthy tissue and histological examination.

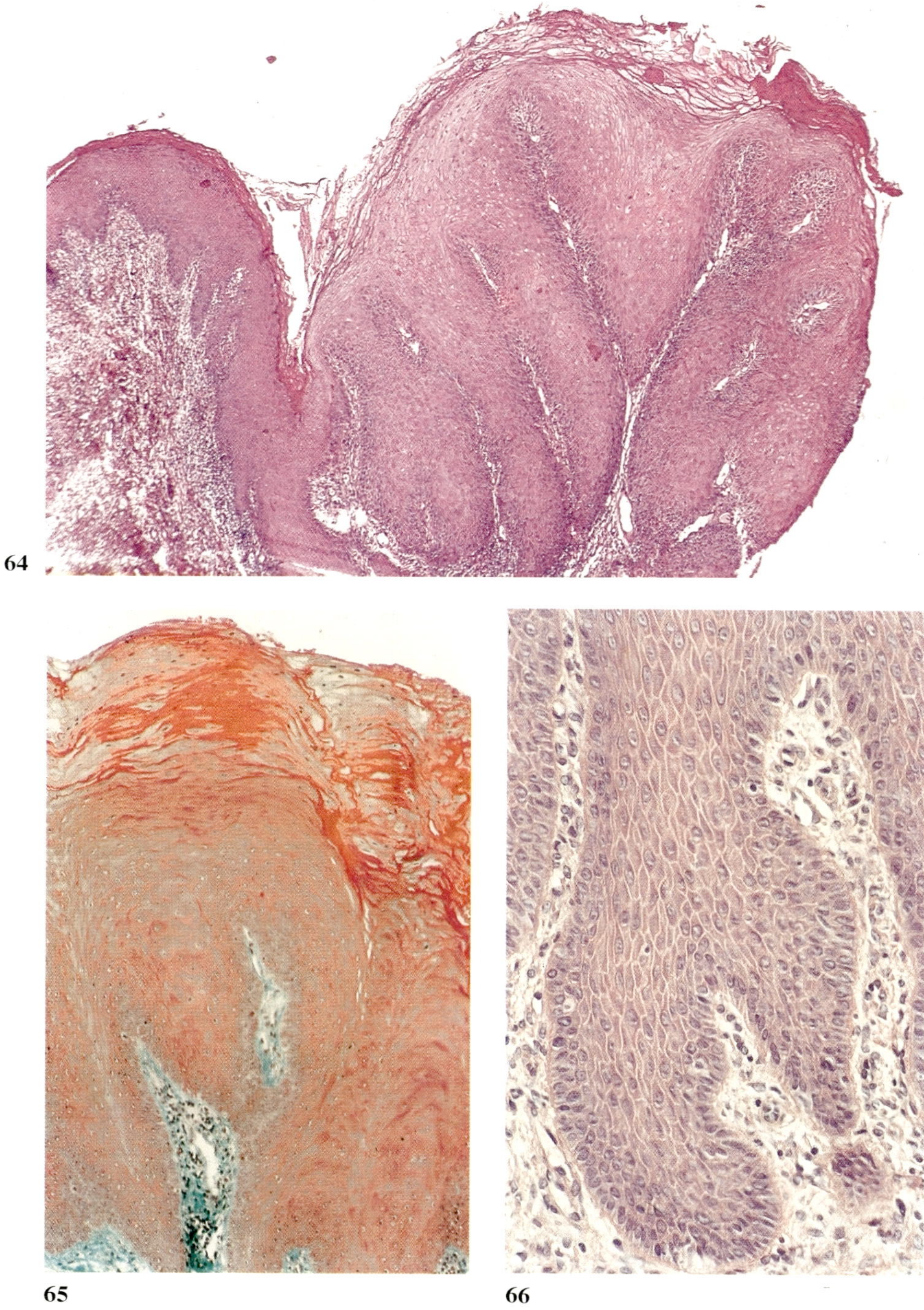

64

65

66

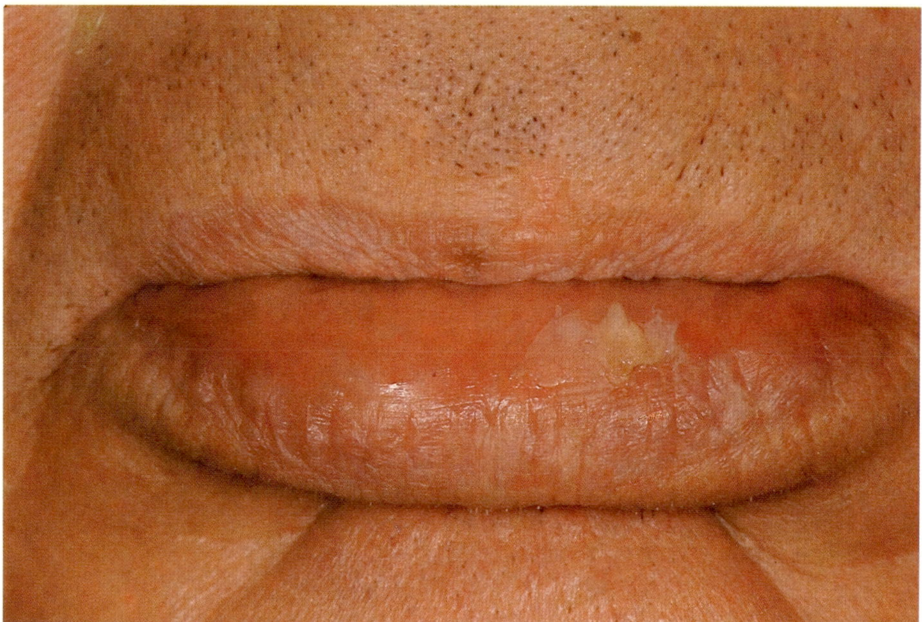

67

67 Fine, whitish-yellow discoloration, that cannot be rubbed off, of transitional epithelium in the region of the lower lip, thickened at the centre. (Male aged 63, pipe smoker; clinically non-suspect)

68 Superficially planar stratified epithelium, with stratification showing only minor changes. Basal cell layer stands out clearly. Prickle cell layer is narrow and superficial to it there is an extensive orthokeratotic horny layer. Increased round cell infiltration can be seen subepithelially. Underlying connective tissue shows 'elastoid' degeneration: collagen fibres are stained a homogeneous red, and react to special stains in the same way as elastic tissue.

69 Rete peg showing marked basal cell dysplasia, with the polar arrangement lost.

70 Detail from basal part of epithelium showing irregular basal cell dysplasia. Nuclei vary in size, in part taking excessive stain. There is an increased number of mitoses, and sub-epithelially round cell infiltrates are present.

Clinical management

Despite the fact that the condition appears harmless clinically, if risk-factors cannot be eliminated (very keen pipe-smoker) excision is indicated to determine the degree of dysplasia. In this case (Figures **67** to **70**), there is a moderate degree of dysplasia. Following total excision, follow-up as part of general treatment programme.

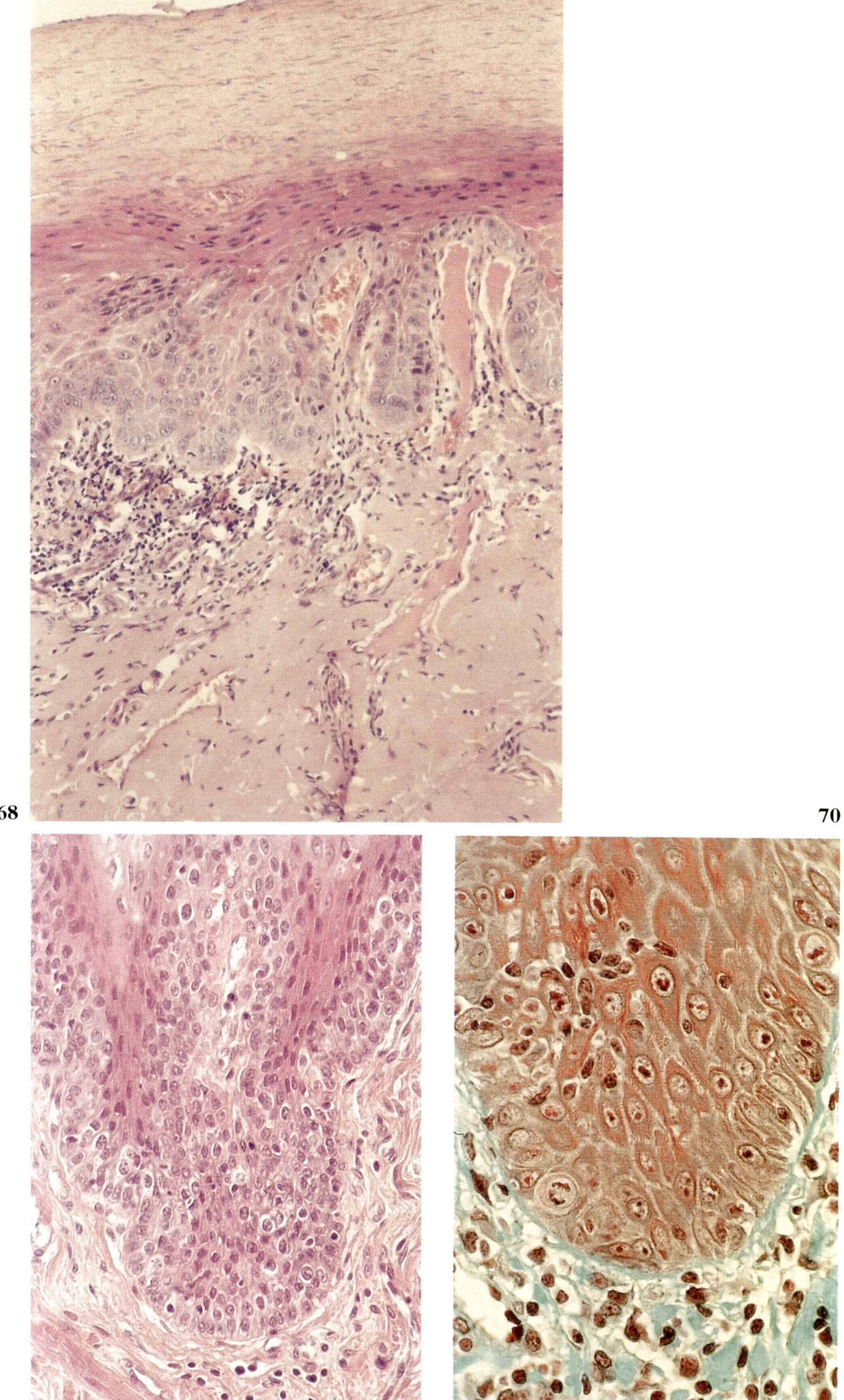
68

70

69

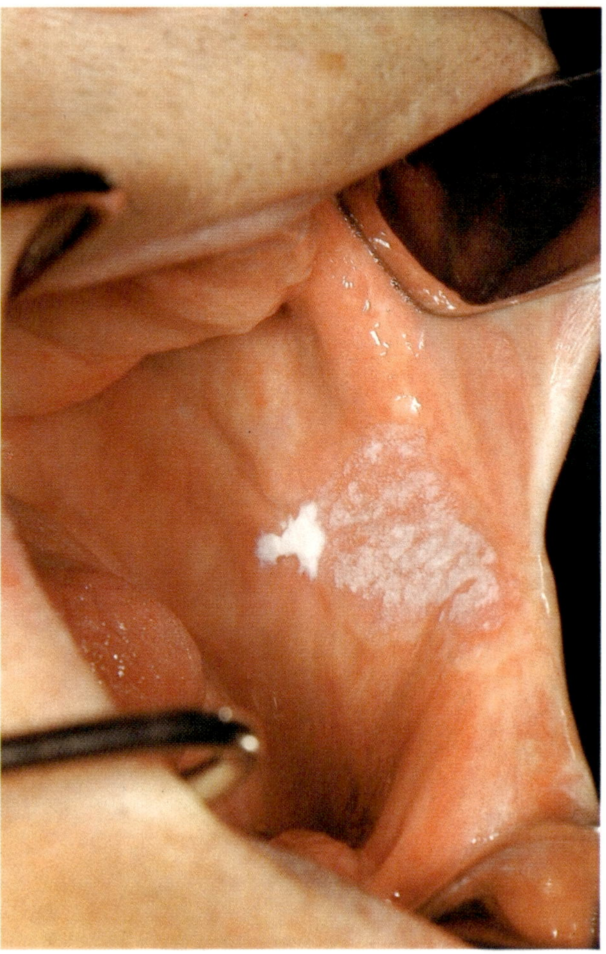

71

71 Immediately retroangular, triangular whitish patches on mucosa that cannot be rubbed off. Surface is irregular, slightly nodular, and depth of coloration is variable. (Male aged 68, denture-wearer and smoker; clinically a precancerous lesion suspected)

72 Planar epithelium with stratification maintained. The basal cell layer is restless and there is marked acanthosis. Superficially is a wide area of hyperorthokeratosis. Increased numbers of round cells are present in connective tissue.

73 Irregular widening of basal cell layer with polar arrangement not discernible. Minor degree of nuclear polymorphism evident.

74 In the lower part of the spinous layer a single rounded, prematurely keratinised cell is clearly discernible (dyskeratosis).

Clinical management

Total excision and histological examination are required. Further measures depend on the degree of dysplasia. In this case (Figures **71** to **74**), there is a moderate degree of dysplasia. Follow-up observation should be undertaken as part of general treatment programme.

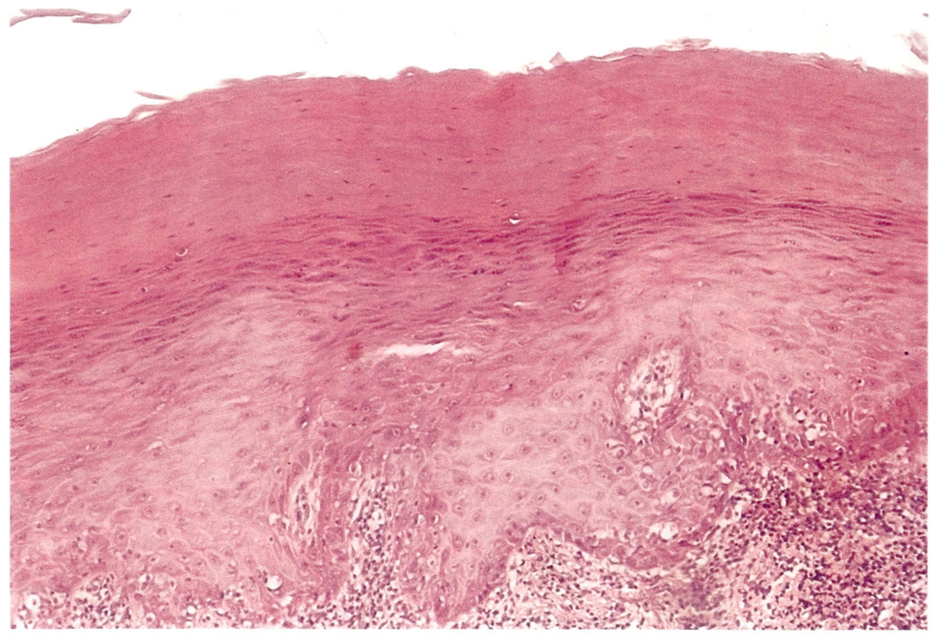

72

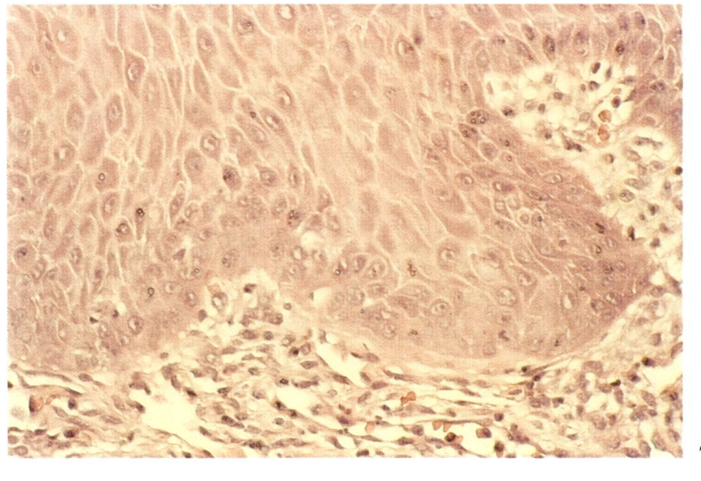

73

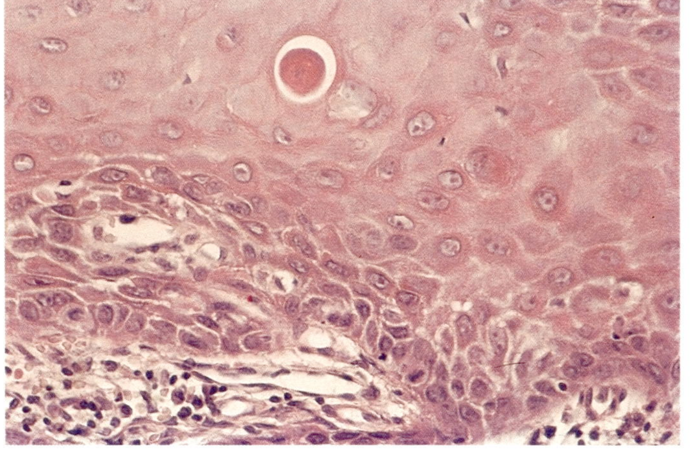

74

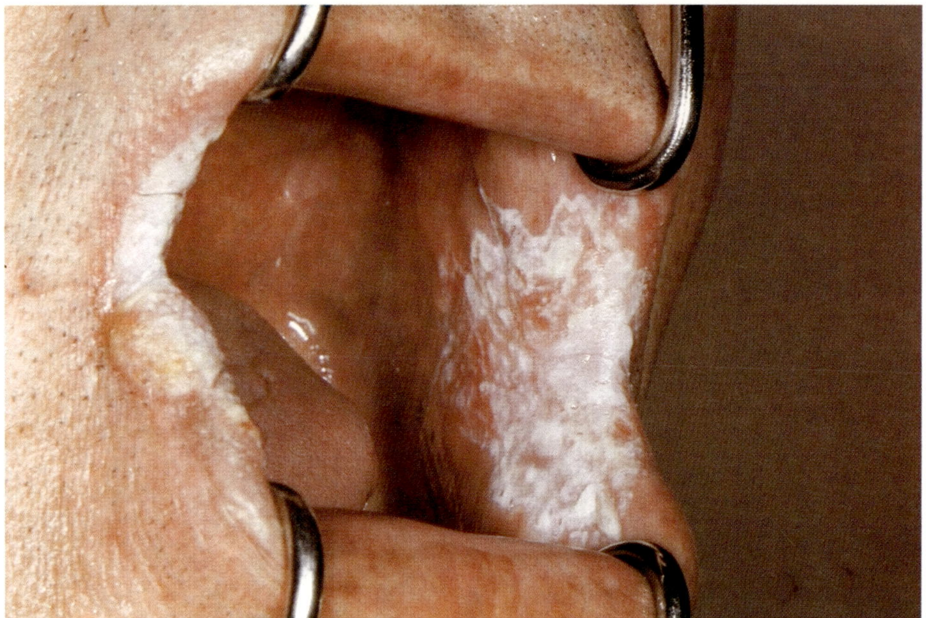

75

75 Whitish mucosal change, that cannot be rubbed off, in the right angle of the mouth and on right buccal surface, with indistinct margins and nodular surface. Verrucous hypertrophic areas alternate with shallow dark-red erosions. A similar change can be seen in the region of the left buccal mucosa and on the external surface of the lip-red in the region of the angle of the mouth, where compact nodular growth, 8 × 10mm in size, is infiltrating the surrounding area ('leukoplakia carcinoma'). (Male aged 56, pipe smoker; highly suggestive of carcinoma on both sides)

Clinical management

Admission to hospital.
Right side: Total excision into healthy tissue and histological examination of fast-frozen section should be performed. Although no carcinoma is found in this case, there is a high degree of dysplasia. Therefore, follow up as for carcinoma (every four weeks for the first year), by specialists of the hospital.
Left side: Excision of nodular lesion into healthy tissue and examination of fast-frozen section should be done. An invasive carcinoma is present, therefore immediate total removal of the angle of the mouth is necessary together with clearance of regional lymph drainage routes. Close follow-up supervision is essential.

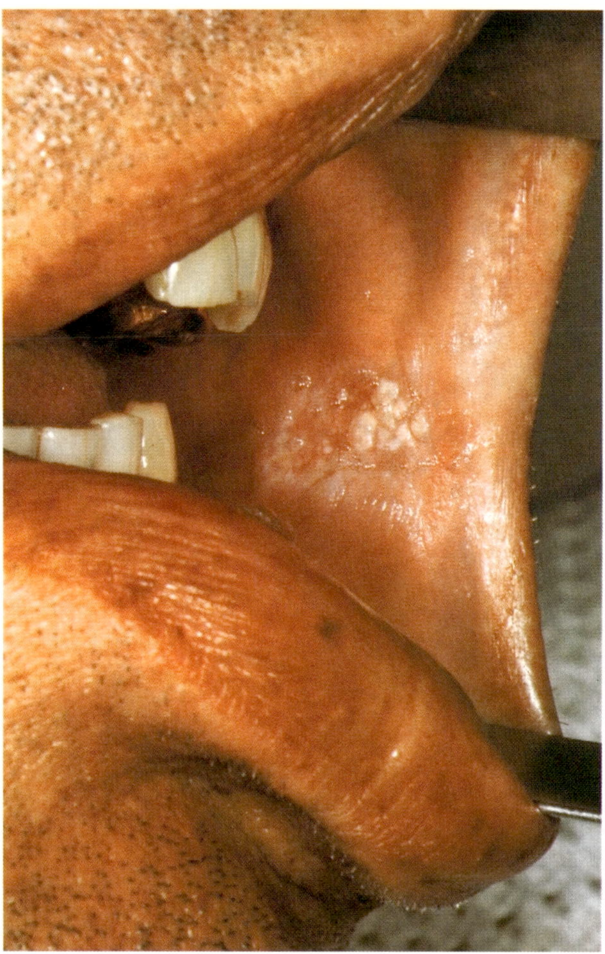

82

82 Retroangular and in the region of the intercalary line of the left buccal mucosa is an erosive mucosal lesion, partly whitish but predominantly red, with a slight degree of marginal infiltration. (Male aged 53, smoker; clinically malignancy suspected)

Clinical management

Admission to hospital for total excision into healthy tissue and histological examination based on fast-frozen section. Although no carcinoma discovered, the high degree of dysplasia does, however, indicate follow-up as for carcinoma in the oncological clinic of the hospital.

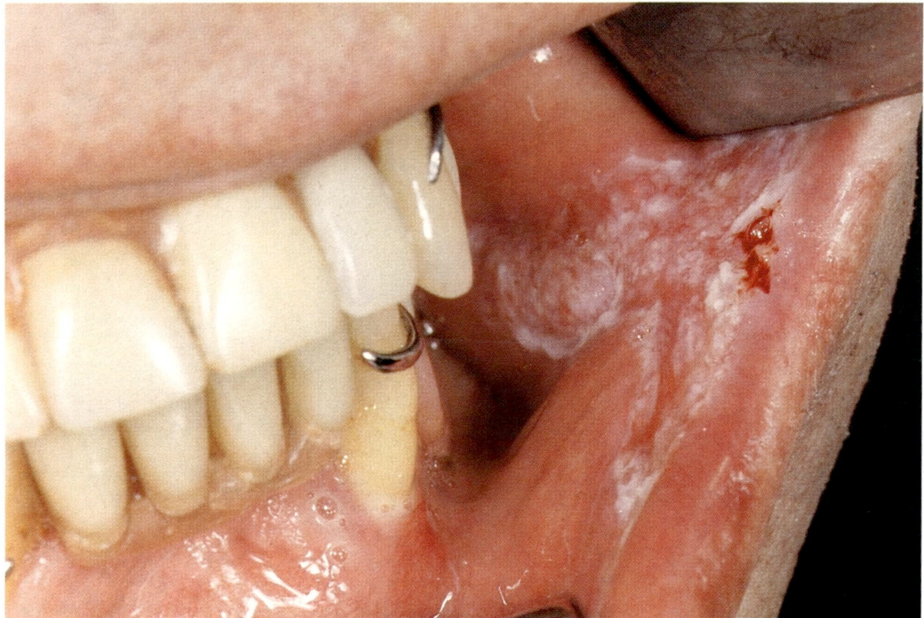

87

87 Extensive white and reddish spotted lesion in the mucosa lining the left cheek, with erosions at the angle of the mouth, in a patient wearing dentures and maintaining poor oral hygiene. There is no infiltration. (Male aged 59, smoker; clinically, a precancerous lesion suspected)

88 Endophytic epithelium, with normal stratification and rete pegs increased in number and size. The basal cell layer is enlarged, with low-degree polymorphism. Superficially, there is extensive hyperparakeratosis, with fungal hyphae clearly discernible, most of them at right angles to the horny squames. Dense inflammatory infiltration can be seen subepithelially.

89 Part of an epithelial rete peg showing basal cell hyperplasia, inflammatory infiltration with round cells and occasional granulocytes. Epithelial stratification also shows abnormalities, with organoid dyskeratosis developing.

Clinical management

Admission to hospital, for immediate biopsy with fast-frozen section to determine surgical procedure. As no carcinoma is discovered, the mucosal lesion only is excised into healthy tissue. The final diagnosis was moderate-degree dysplasia with *Candida albicans* infection. Antimycotic therapy should be given, with close follow-up observation.

88

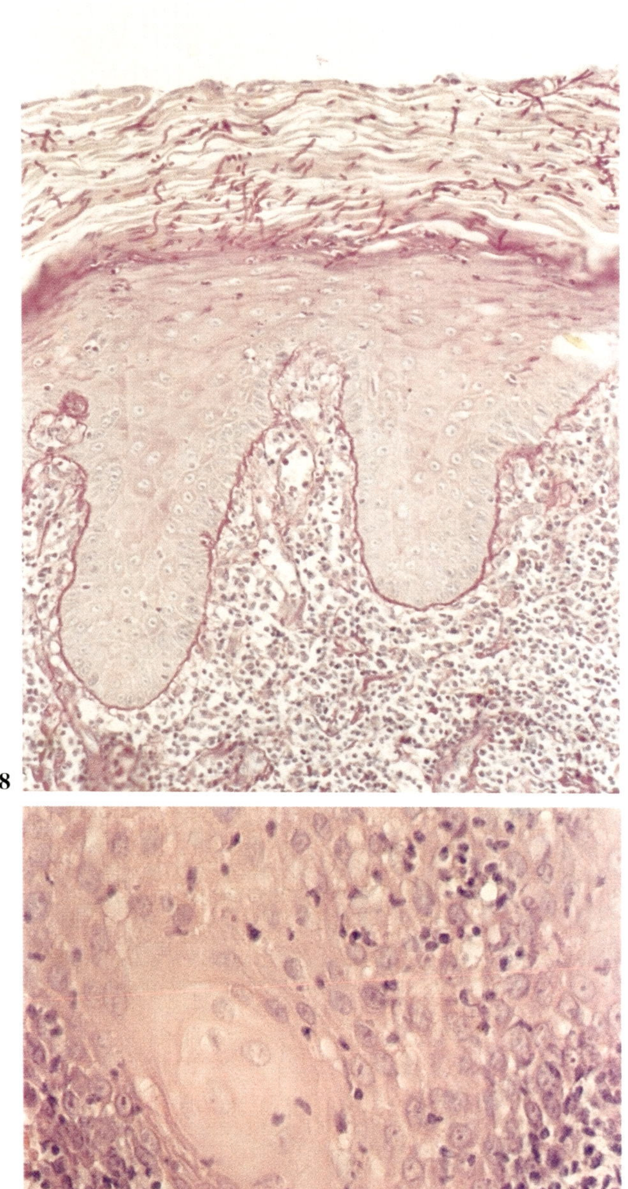

89

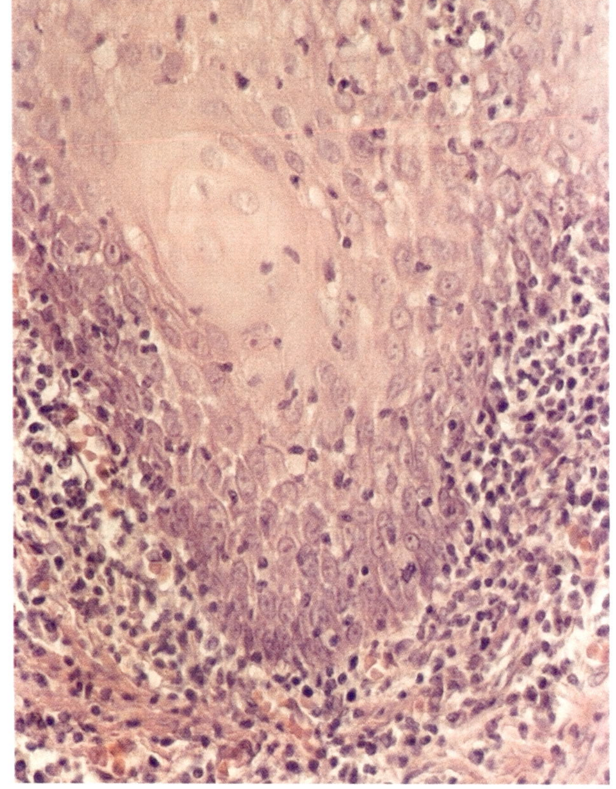

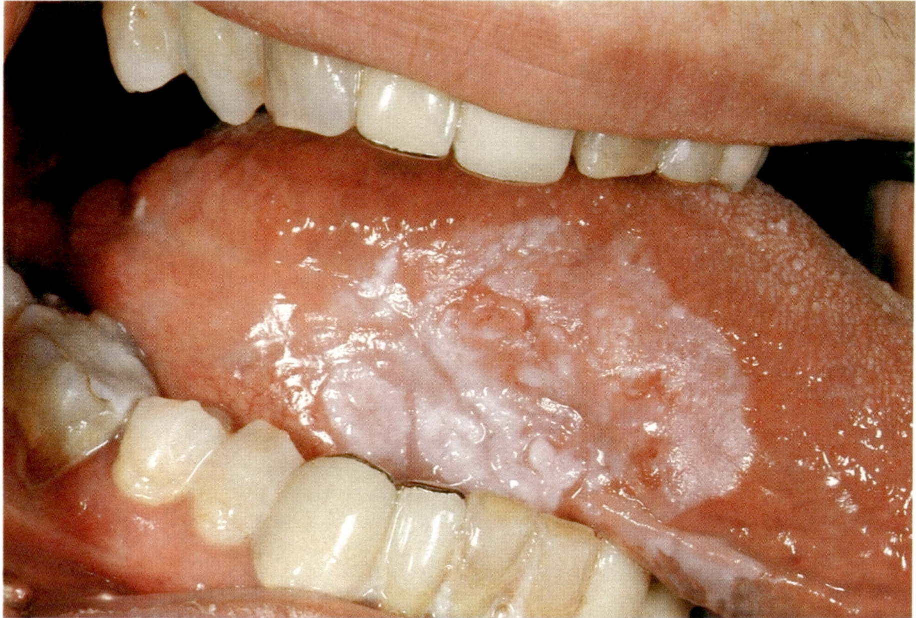

90

90 Extensive whitish lesion in the mucosa of the tongue that cannot be rubbed off. Some parts are verrucous, while the centre is reddish and erosive. There is no infiltration. (Female aged 71; clinically, a precancerous lesion suspected)

91 Endophytic epithelium with very marked basal rete pegs. Considerable basal cell hyperplasia is present in this area, with cellular polymorphism. The prickle cell layer has broadened with intracellular glycogen demonstrable occasionally. Superficially, there is dense fungal growth with hyphae selectively stained. *(PAS)*

92 Detail of superficial strata of epithelium. Horny squames show dense granulocytic infiltration. Fungal hyphae are not shown up by this stain. *(H&E)*

93 Fungal hyphae stained bright red. *(PAS)*

Clinical management

Admission to hospital. Biopsy only should be taken at first to determine surgical procedure, and a fast-frozen section examined histologically. As no carcinoma was found only resection of affected mucosa from the edge of the tongue into healthy tissue should be performed. The final diagnosis was moderate-degree dysplasia with *Candida albicans* infection. Treatment involves antimycotic therapy and, in view of the risk-factor associated with the location and because of the fungus infection, close follow-up observation.

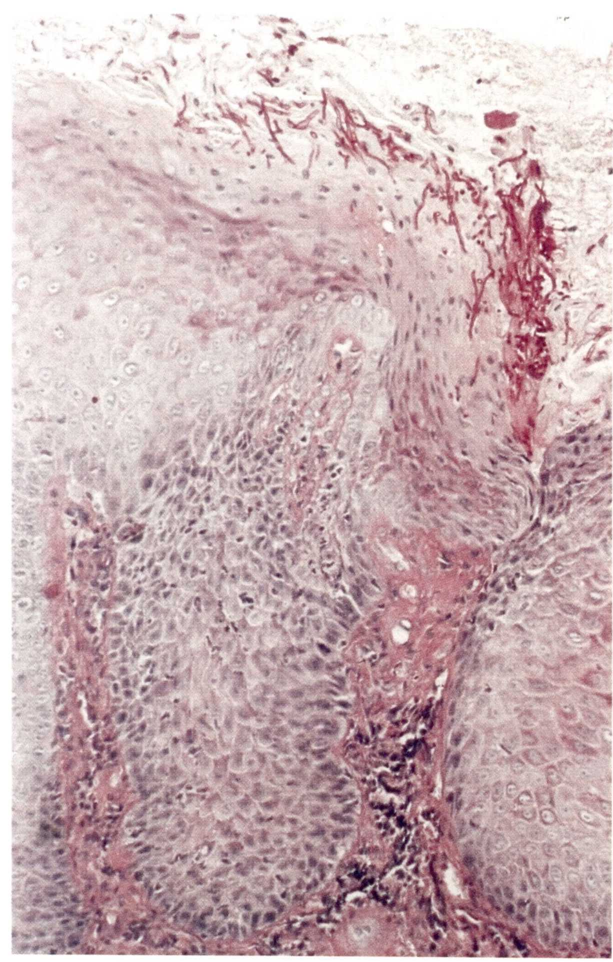

91

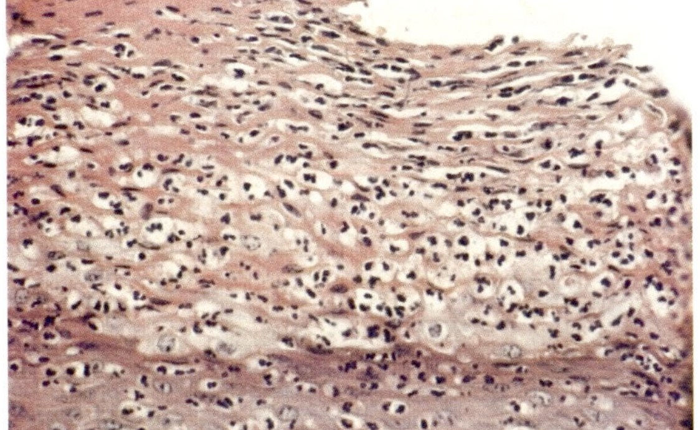

92

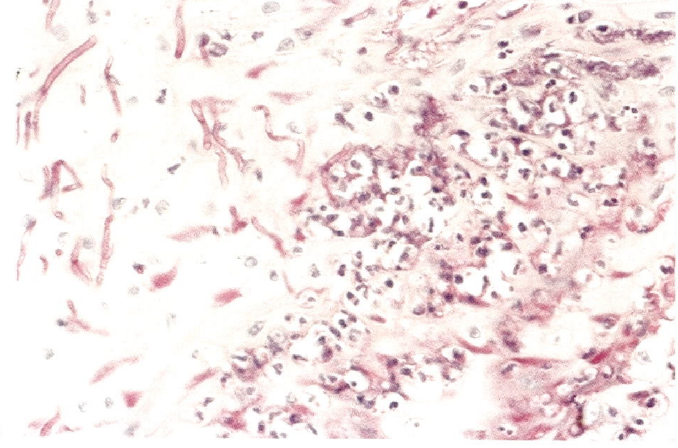

93

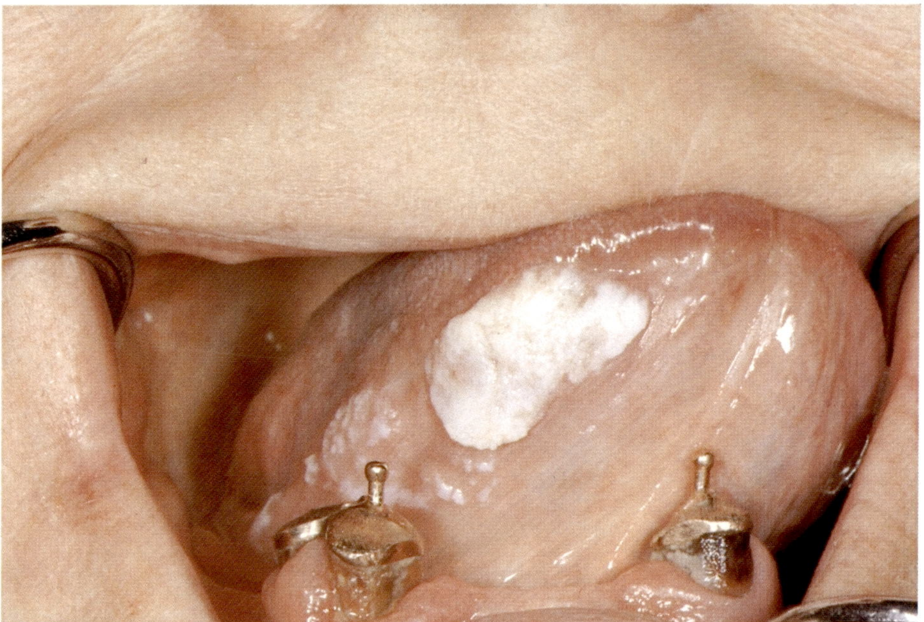

94

94 A thick, hard, raised, clearly circumscribed whitish lesion, that does not rub off, in the mucosa of the tongue. Concurrently distal to this are further whitish nodular changes in the mucosa. (Female aged 67; precancerous lesion suspected)

95 Marked epithelial hyperplasia (centre), abrupt and with definite acanthosis.

96 Epithelial rete peg showing somewhat restless basal cell hyperplasia, though polar arrangement is still discernible. Round cell infiltrate can be seen sub-epithelially.

Clinical management

Excision into healthy tissue, and determination of degree of dysplasia should be performed. In this case, there is a moderate degree of dysplasia. As the location carries a risk-factor, total removal is necessary with follow-up at regular intervals.

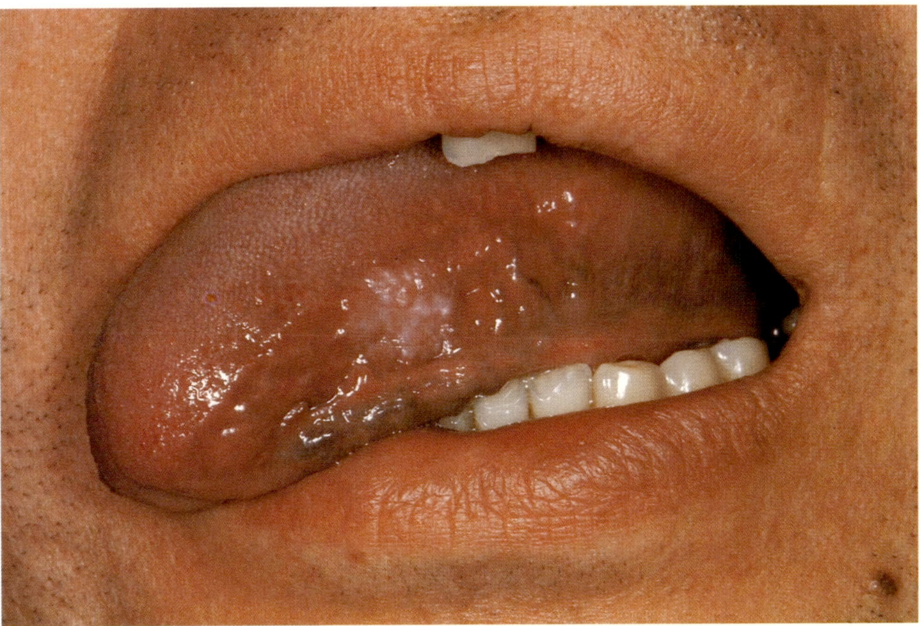

99

99 Whitish and pale pink discoloration, 1 × 1cm in area and not hypertrophic, in the mucosa at the margin of the tongue. No infiltration. (Male aged 31; clinically, a precancerous lesion suspected)

100 Highly endophytic epithelium showing a marked increase in disordered basal rete peg formation. Basal cells are definitely increased and fibrosis of subepithelial stroma is evident. Immediately inferior to the epithelium, there is loosening of connective tissue, with occasional round cell infiltrates.

101 Detail of epithelial rete peg showing restless basal cell hyperplasia and a minor degree of cellular polymorphism. Prickle cells show irregular staining indicative of abnormal differentiation with variable tonofibril content. Increased numbers of interepithelial cells are present.

102 Basal epithelial rete peg showing marked cellular polymorphism and nuclear hyperchromatism. Increased and ectatic capillaries can be seen immediately inferior to the epithelium, possibly due to angiogenetic substances produced in the dysplastic epithelium.

Clinical management

Total excision into healthy tissue and determination of degree of dysplasia should be carried out. In this case there is a moderate degree of dysplasia. Risk-factor of location necessitates regular follow-up observation.

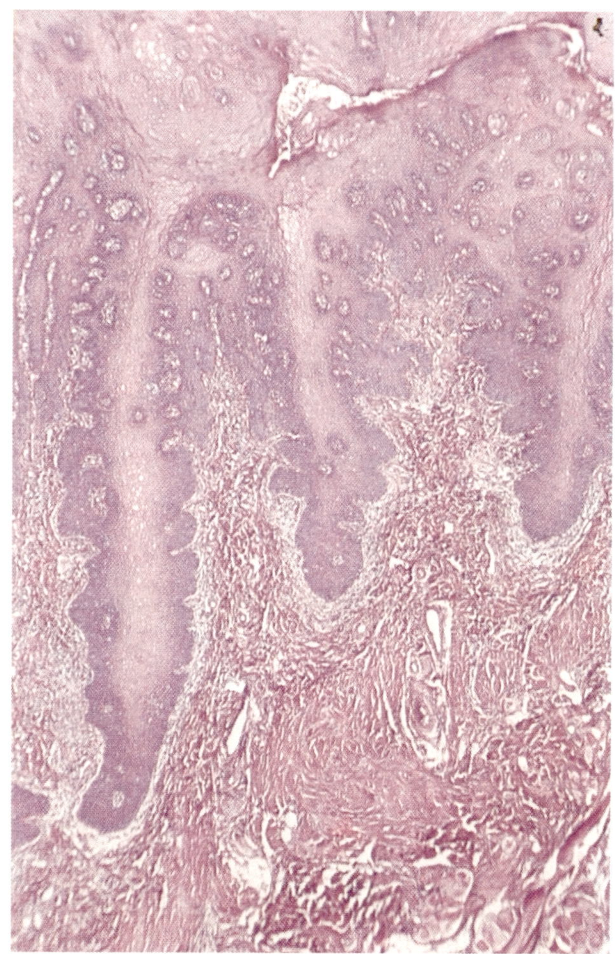

100

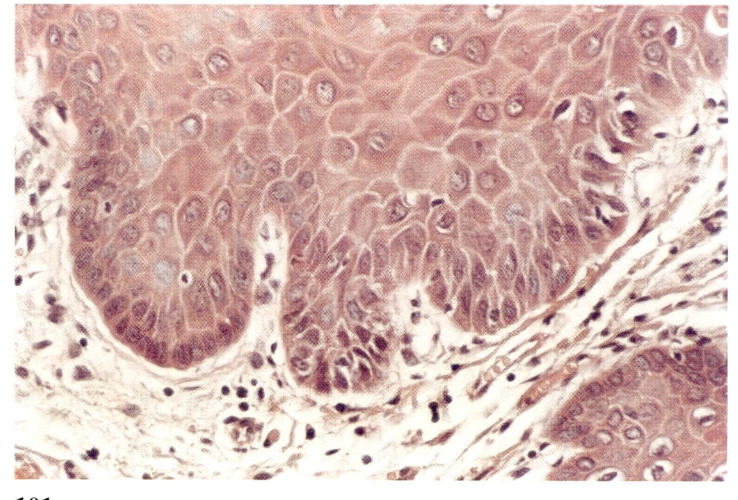

101

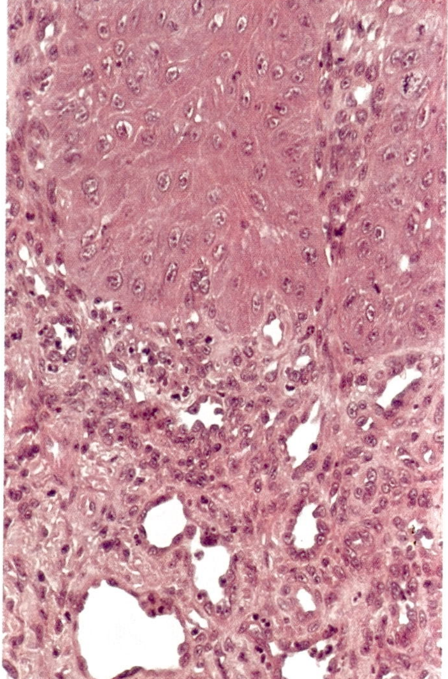

102

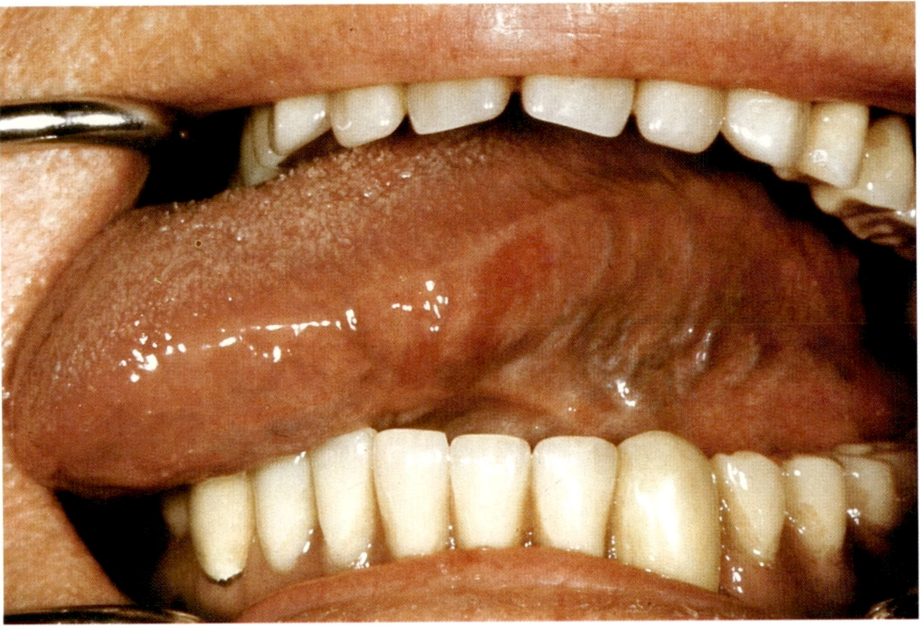

103

103 Raspberry-red lesion in mucosa at margin of tongue showing slight degree of marginal infiltration. (Female aged 65; clinically, high suspicion of malignancy)

104 Epithelium showing total loss of stratification. A basal cell layer cannot be defined and cohesion is broken, resulting in interepithelial spaces. Marked hyperchromatism and nuclear polymorphism are evident.

105 Focal epithelial atrophy, with squamous cornification merely indicated on the right side of the picture, and marked cellular and nuclear polymorphism.

106 Highly dysplastic, sometimes fusiform, irregularly arranged cell formations in the region of the basal cell and prickle cell layers.

Clinical management

Admission to hospital for total excision and fast-frozen section for histological examination. In this case (Figures **103** to **106**), no invasive carcinoma was found. Examination of paraffin-embedded material showed carcinoma *in situ*. Follow-up observation as for invasive carcinoma is therefore necessary, in the oncological clinic of the hospital.

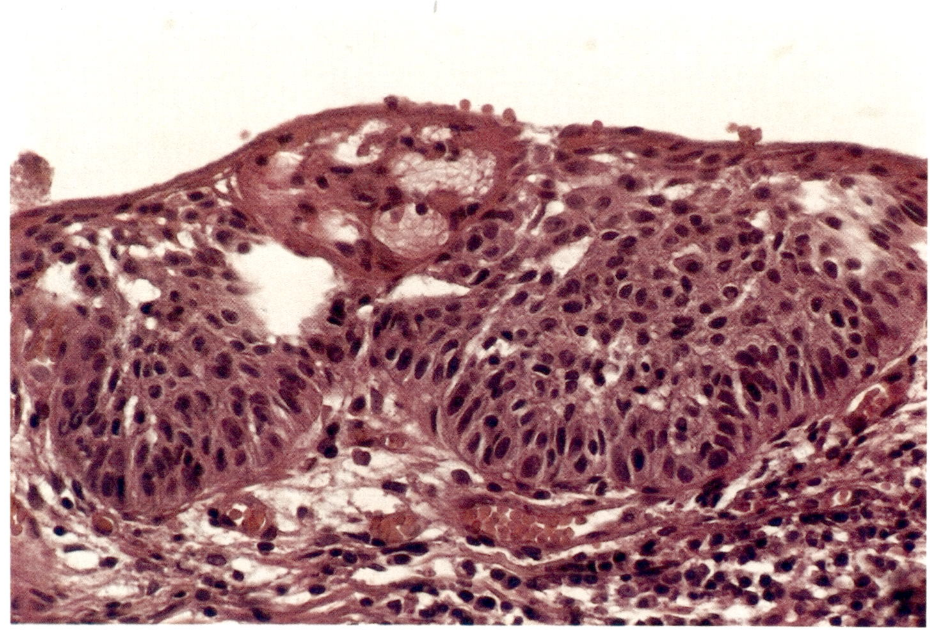

104

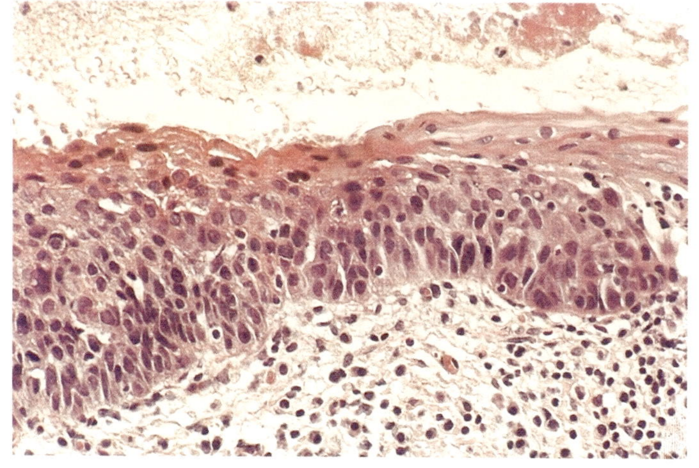

105

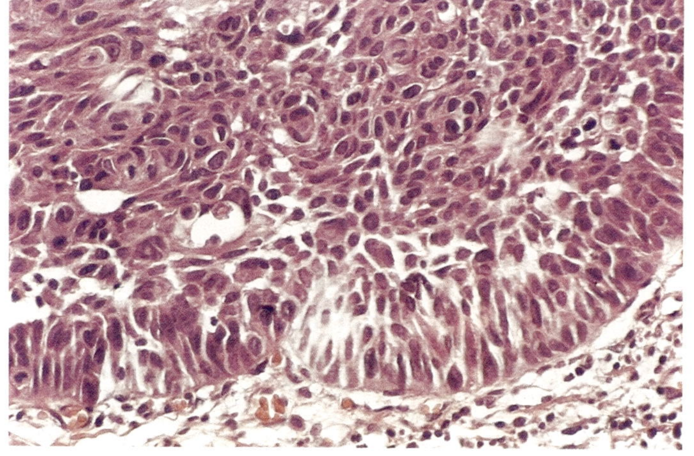

106

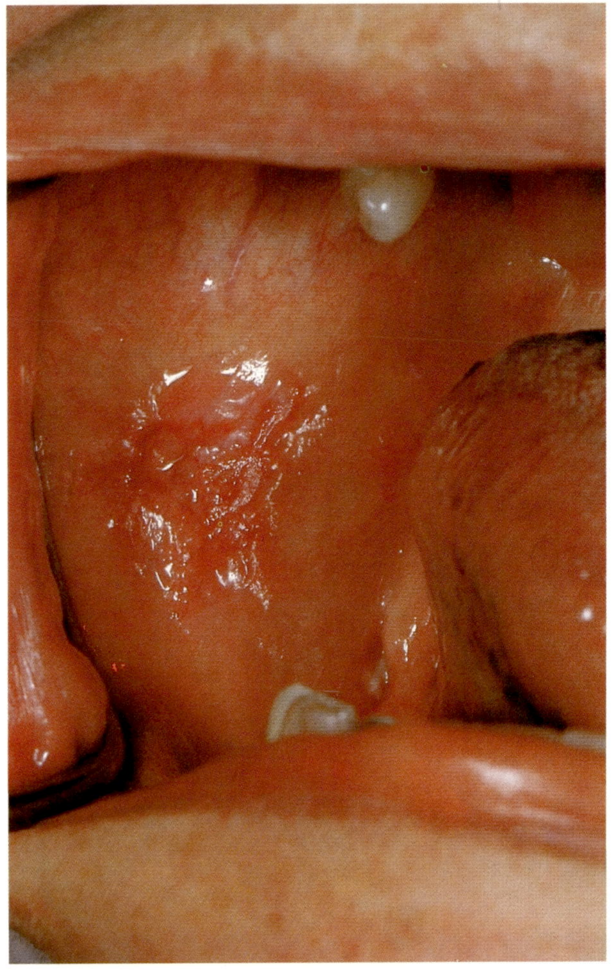

107

107 Dark-red discoloration of mucosa, 2 × 2cm in area, in the posterior part of the buccal surface. There is a minor degree of marginal infiltration, but no deep ulceration. (Female aged 74; clinically, high suspicion of malignancy)

108 Thickness of epithelium definitely increased, with considerable disorganisation of stratification. Small, fusiform cell formations, showing nuclear hyperchromatism and considerable cellular polymorphism, occupy almost the whole thickness of epithelium. Only in the superficial parts of the epithelium are single rows of prickle cell-like cells, with a thin layer of flattened cells at the surface.

109 High magnification of basal parts of epithelium reveals densely packed cells, predominantly fusiform, with hyperchromatic and polymorphic nuclei. There is a dense round cell stroma reaction subepithelially.

110 Densely packed lymphocytes and plasma cells in the subepithelial stroma and brilliant red Russell bodies. *(PAS)*

Clinical management

Admission to hospital for total excision and examination of fast-frozen section. In this case (Figures **107** to **110**), no invasive carcinoma was found. Examination of paraffin-embedded material showed carcinoma *in situ*. Follow-up observation as for invasive carcinoma is therefore required, in the oncological clinic of the hospital.

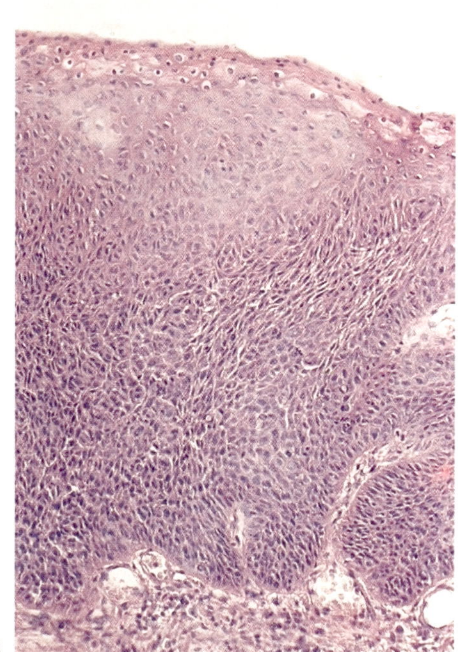

108

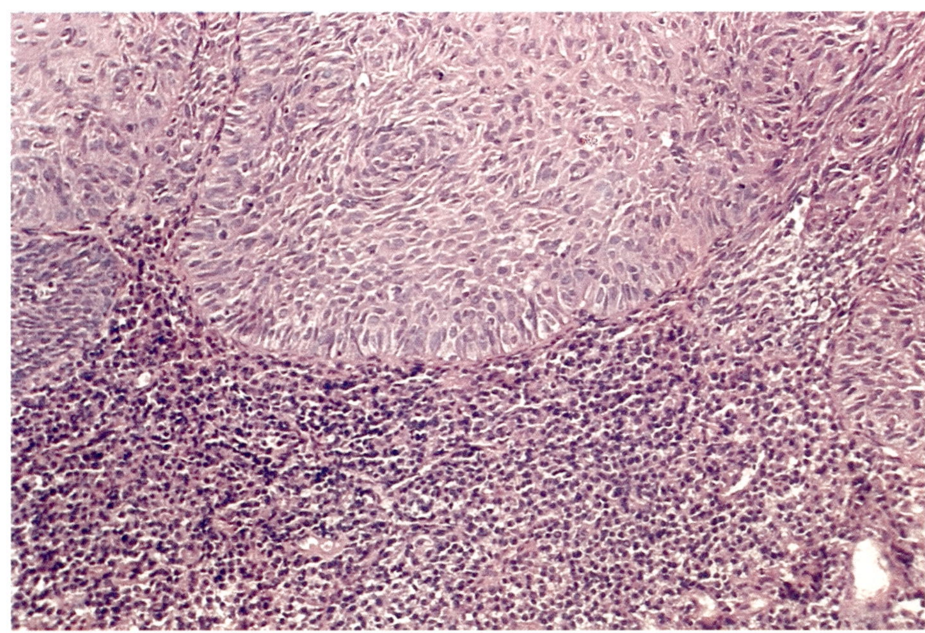

109

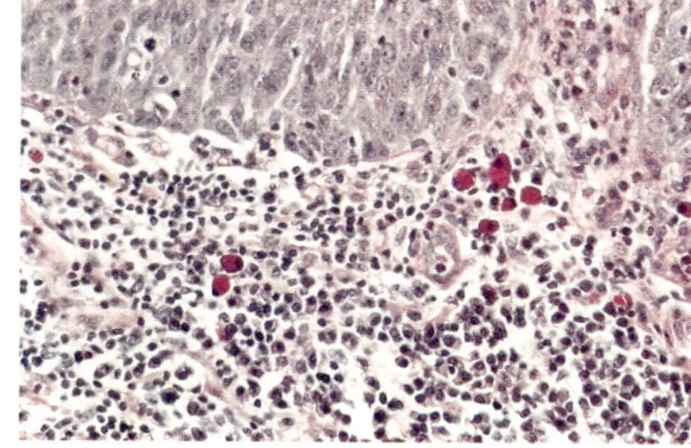

110

Differentiation based on tissue studies, *i.e.* the degree of dysplasia, forms the basis for a differential treatment and follow-up plan appropriate to stage (Tables 9 to 11). If different tissue samples show different degrees of dysplasia, clinical management will be based on the *highest* degree of dysplasia. Where risk-factors cannot be eliminated (tobacco or alcohol abuse), lesions appear particularly suspect clinically (erosive leukoplakia, erythroplakia), or are located in high-risk areas (tongue and floor of the mouth) and in cases of fungus infection, the procedures relating to the *second highest* stage should be adopted. *Candida* infection requires antimycotic therapy in addition. Patients should always be instructed to monitor this for themselves.

Table 9 Clinical Management with a Diagnosis of No Epithelial Dysplasia or Low-Degree Dysplasia

No/low-degree dysplasia
– aim at total excision
– if excision total, no follow-up observation
– if excision incomplete, further observation at longer intervals (3–6 months)

Table 10 Clinical Management with a Diagnosis of Medium-Degree Epithelial Dysplasia

Medium-degree dysplasia
– aim for total excision
– if removal incomplete initially, total excision to follow
– with total excision, no follow-up observation
– if excision incomplete, further observation at shorter intervals (4–8 weeks)

Table 11 Clinical Management with a Diagnosis of Marked Dysplasia and with Carcinoma *in situ*

Marked dysplasia (and carcinoma *in situ*)
– total excision in every case
– follow-up as for cancer patients (every 4 weeks during the first year)

4 Early stages of cancer and dissimulating cancers (carcinoma dissimulans)

Clinical features

The early diagnosis of manifest carcinoma in the oral cavity tends to be a problem because there are no truly specific early symptoms. Following onset of invasive growth, oral cancer goes through an asymptomatic early stage of varying duration, and may still present as a precancerous condition, such as leukoplakia or erythroplakia. Tumours presenting as leukoplakia are also referred to as leukoplakia carcinomata. A more common feature at this stage, however, are reddish changes and small ulcerated lesions in the mucosa. Carcinomata masked by the symptoms and signs of precancer, or of benign mucosal lesions in the oral cavity, are a particular diagnostic problem. They may be usefully referred to as dissimulating carcinomata (carcinoma dissimulans). We use this term to describe a carcinoma that is usually only small in size, clinically symptom-free, or presenting with only few symptoms, and frequently misdiagnosed on the basis of its macroscopic appearance.

Unfortunately, experience has frequently shown that even tumours showing only a slight degree of invasive growth may already have produced metastatic growth in the regional lymph nodes. This applies particularly to cancers located in the floor of the mouth and in the tongue. Major factors contributing to this situation are that these parts of the oral mucosa are particularly well supplied with lymph vessels, and also the absence of a tunica muscularis mucosae delimiting the lamina propria. For this reason pathological anatomy offers no definition for early carcinoma of the oral cavity based on depth of infiltration or invasion beyond the tunica muscularis, such as is used, for instance, in the region of the gastric mucosa.

Larger tumours may show more exophytic and papillomatous growth or be nodular and endophytic. In the latter case, ulceration of the mucosa is the rule.

Apart from inspection, palpation is an essential requirement for assessing a lesion in the mucosa. Carcinomata will frequently show noticeable marginal infiltration in the initial stages. Symptoms will usually appear only at an advanced stage, so that medical help is frequently sought too late. In order of frequency these symptoms are:

1 Irritation of mucosa due to more deep-reaching ulceration
2 Spontaneous bleeding from the mucosa
3 Extensive indurations
4 Pain
5 Loosening of teeth

Histopathology

Due to their origin in stratified squamous epithelium, oral carcinomata generally present as a squamous cell carcinoma. Other forms of cancer are rare (adenocarcinoma, adenoid cystic carcinoma) and arise from the small salivary glands. Keratinising squamous cell carcinoma is the most common form of differentiation; non-keratinising carcinomata, anaplastic carcinomata, and mixed forms – partly basal cell and partly prickle cell carcinoma – are uncommon.

Histological diagnosis of advanced carcinoma is not difficult as a rule, but problems may arise with early invasive cancer. Tangential and transverse sections through rete pegs may wrongly suggest cell complexes 'dropping off'. Diagnosis is assisted by visualisation of the basement membrane (PAS staining, silvering), and it is also important to consider the total architectural composition as well as cellular dysplasia or atypia.

Like leukoplakia, squamous cell carcinoma of the oral cavity is not uniform in biological significance, and this is taken into account when establishing the degree of malignancy, by grading tumours as I (highly differentiated) to IV (anaplastic). Grading is based on the estimated ratio of differentiated to undifferentiated elements in the tumour. Grade I indicates a ratio of 100 to 75 per cent differentiated to 0 to 25 per cent undifferentiated elements, Grade II a ratio of 75 to 50 per cent to 25 to 50 per cent, Grade III one of 50 to 25 per cent to 50 to 75 per cent, and Grade IV one of 25 to 0 per cent differentiated to 75 to 100 per cent undifferentiated elements. Oral cancers are also quite frequently classified according to three degrees of differentiation (well, medium, poorly). A division into degrees of anaplasia or atypia (low, medium and high) would seem more appropriate, as these correspond directly to the degrees of dysplasia seen in precancerous conditions. Determining the degrees of malignancy in this way presents a number of problems. Tumours may show variable differentiation, and a small amount of biopsy material is not always representative of the whole tumour. Grading has little bearing on prognosis and treatment, as these are also determined by a considerable number of other factors (*e.g.* size, location, prior treatment, immune status). Highly differentiated tumours do, however, have a better prognosis on the whole, and also respond better to cytostatic treatment with bleomycin.

Apart from 'ordinary' squamous cell carcinoma, two special forms of oral cancer are known – verrucous and spindle cell carcinoma. (Lymphoepithelioma arising in the tonsillar region may be omitted from our considerations.)

Verrucous carcinoma, also known as Ackerman's tumour, presents clinically as a verrucous exophytic tumour with a deeply plicated greyish-white surface. It is frequently associated with leukoplakia. Differential diagnosis is important because of the clinical implications, as this type of tumour shows much slower growth and offers a better prognosis. Neck dissection is not required, as the tumour may produce local invasion and displacement but rarely metastasises. Irradiation may, however, be followed by dedifferentiation and metastasis.

The histology is also quite characteristic. In the margins, abrupt transition into highly hyperplastic epithelium is noted, with exophytic papillomatous projections as well as marked endophytic growth in the form of broad rete pegs and cones. The surface shows a high degree of keratinisation, and typical keratin plugs are found deep down in the rete pegs. Epithelial stratification is on the whole maintained. A characteristic feature is a marked inflammatory reaction in the stroma. Differentiation must be made from papillary endophytic leukoplakia on the one hand, and the highly differentiated squamous cell carcinoma on the other. Verrucous carcinoma is relatively uncommon in the Western world, representing approximately one per cent of oral cancers.

Spindle cell carcinoma of the squamous epithelium in the oral cavity is even less frequently seen than verrucous carcinoma. It represents the opposite extreme to verrucous carcinoma in the scale of differentiation. Primary spindle cell carcinomata also occur as skin tumours and in other parts of the upper digestive and respiratory tracts. They are often polypoid. More common than the primary form are secondary spindle cell carcinomata arising due to transformation of an ordinary squamous cell carcinoma following treatment (irradiation, cytostatics). The histological differentiation of this carcinoma from malignant mesenchymal tumours can present difficulties.

Therapy

It is not our intention to discuss the specific treatment of oral carcinoma. The principle of radical surgery combined with neck dissection as a block operation applies also to the early stages of these cancers. The oral mucosa is richly supplied with lymph vessels, and this may lead to regional metastasisation at the early invasive stage. From this point of view too, therefore, the tongue and the floor of the mouth must be considered high-risk locations.

Chemotherapy now holds a firm place next to radiotherapy in the treatment programme. The antineoplastic agent bleomycin has proved of particular value in the treatment of highly differentiated keratinising squamous cell carcinomata, especially by intra-arterial perfusion of the tumour area.

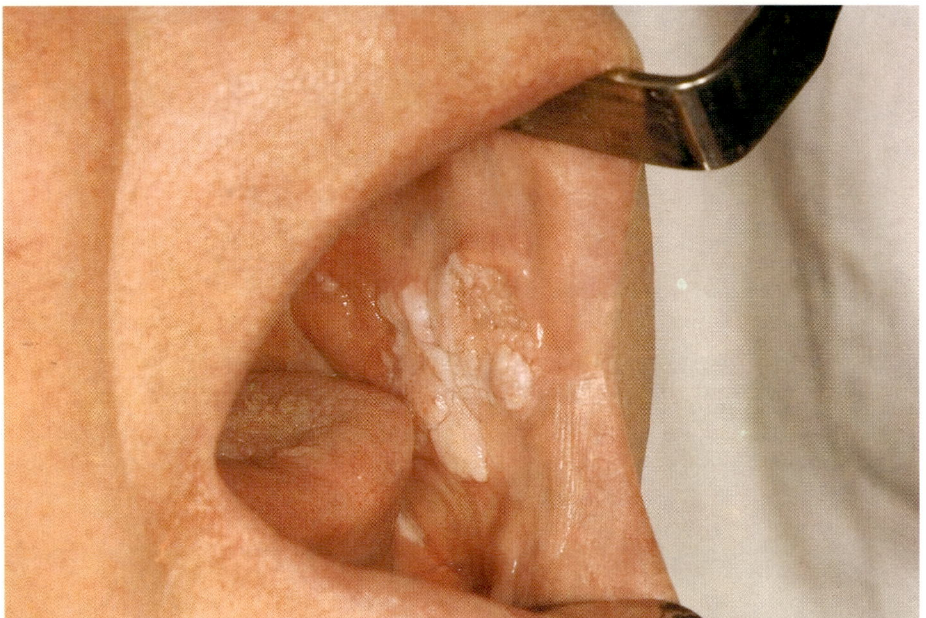

111

111 Extensive planar hypertrophic white lesion in the mucosa, in the region of the left buccal surface, with erosive changes anteriorly. Marginal ridging is clearly discernible in this area. (Male aged 68, heavy smoker; clinically, a carcinoma suspected)

112 Superficially stratified epithelium still shows regular differentiation, with acanthosis and parakeratosis. Inferior to this, polymorphic groups of cells are clearly invasive and occasional epithelial pearls are evident.

113 Strands of tumour cells with marked hyperchromatism and epithelial pearls.

Clinical management

Admission to hospital for histological verification of diagnosis based on fast-frozen section, followed immediately by specific tumour therapy.

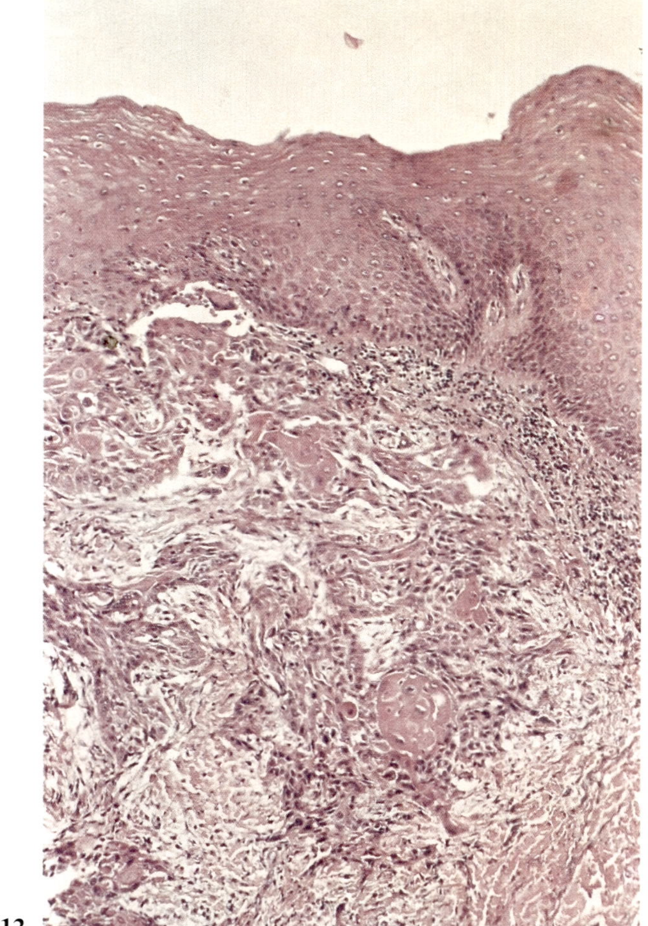

112

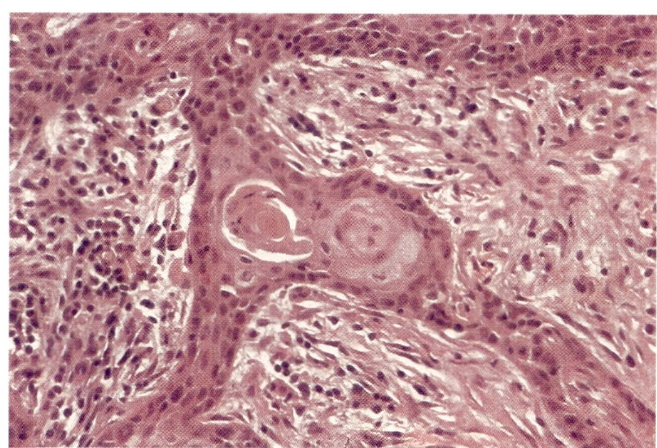

113

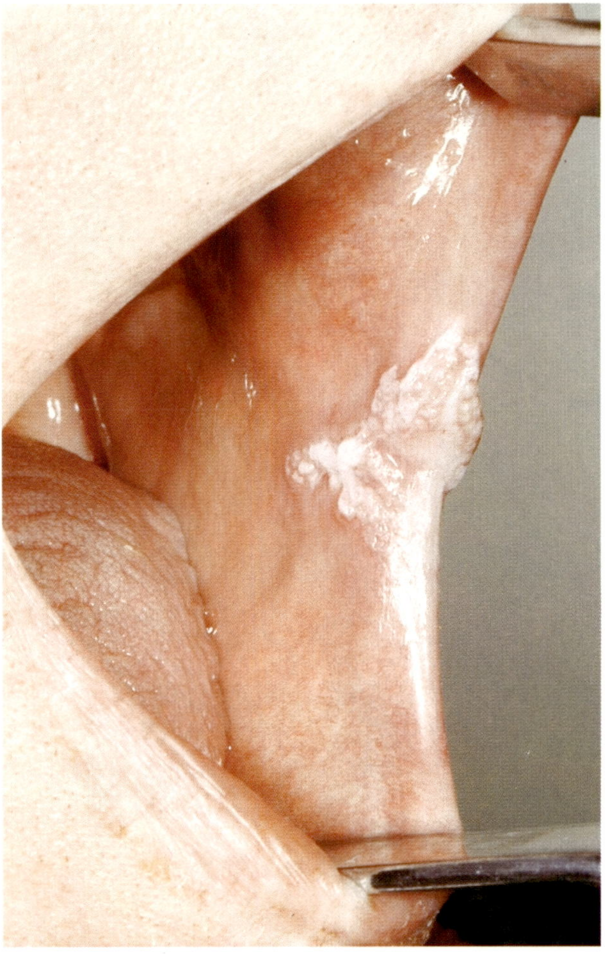

114

114 A nodular, slightly erosive, whitish mucosal lesion above the level of buccal and labial mucosa in the region of the right angle of the mouth. A nodular infiltration is clearly visible and palpable at the centre. (Male aged 55, smoker; clinically, malignancy suspected)

115 Superficially, stratified endophytic epithelium is still extant, with obvious abnormalities of stratification, acanthosis and hyperorthokeratosis. Basal parts show invasive growth of irregular groups of tumour cells into connective tissue (stained green). *(Masson–Goldner)*

116 High magnification of tumour cell cone showing clearly established cellular and nuclear polymorphism and keratinisation, with epithelial pearls (red).

Clinical management

Admission to hospital for resection of angle of mouth and histological examination of fast-frozen section. An invasive carcinoma was found and specific tumour therapy therefore started immediately.

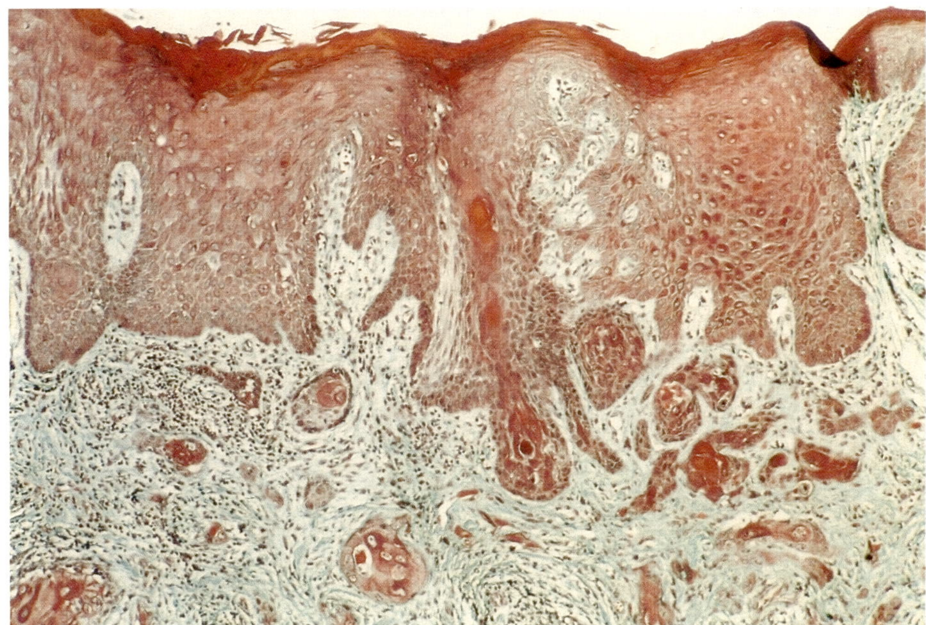
115

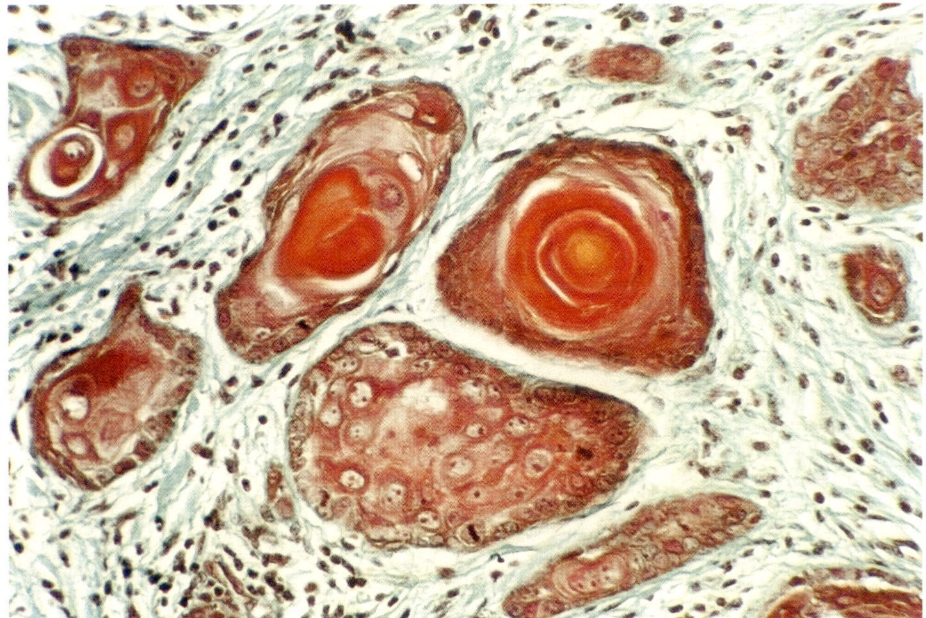
116

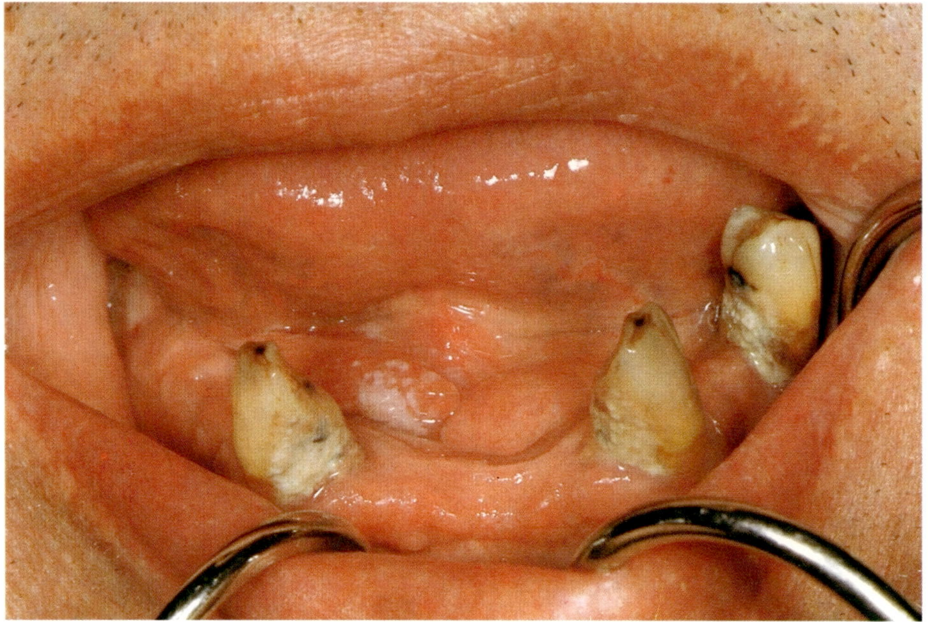

117

117 Immediately above the plica submandibularis a whitish to reddish, slightly verrucous mucosal lesion can be seen, infiltrating surrounding tissues to a minor degree. Residual dentition is not well cared for and shows plaque and dental calculus. (Male aged 71, smoker and alcoholic; clinically, malignancy suspected)

118 Superficially, epithelium shows focal atrophy and hyperorthokeratosis. Basally, occasional epithelial cell groups are 'dropping off', with a high degree of dysplasia. The region also shows a dense round cell reaction in the stroma.

119 High-power micrograph of tumour cell groups showing considerable cellular and nuclear polymorphism, and an area of keratinisation.

Clinical management

Admission to hospital for total excision of the lesion into healthy tissue and examination of fast-frozen section. An early invasive carcinoma was found and specific tumour therapy therefore initiated immediately.

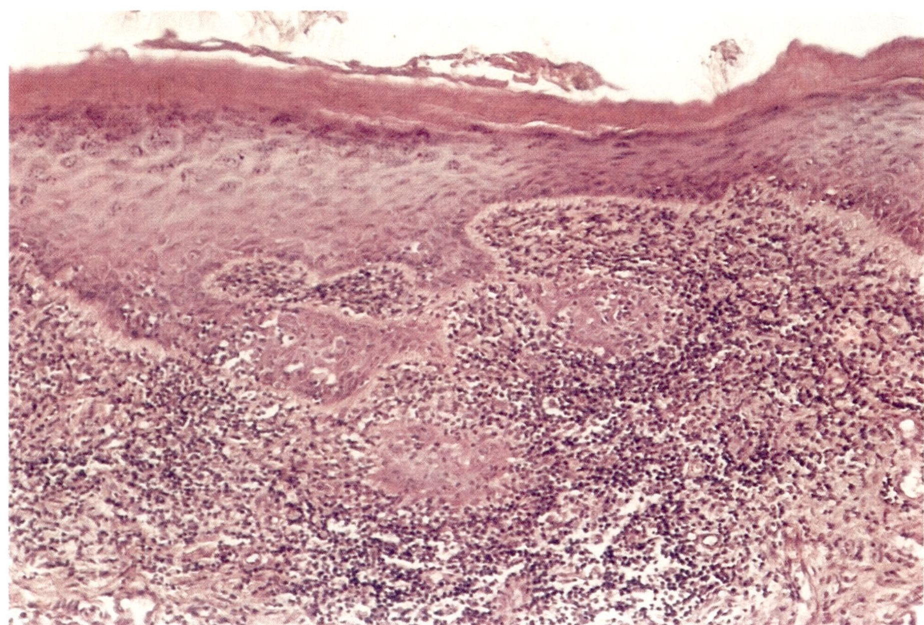
118

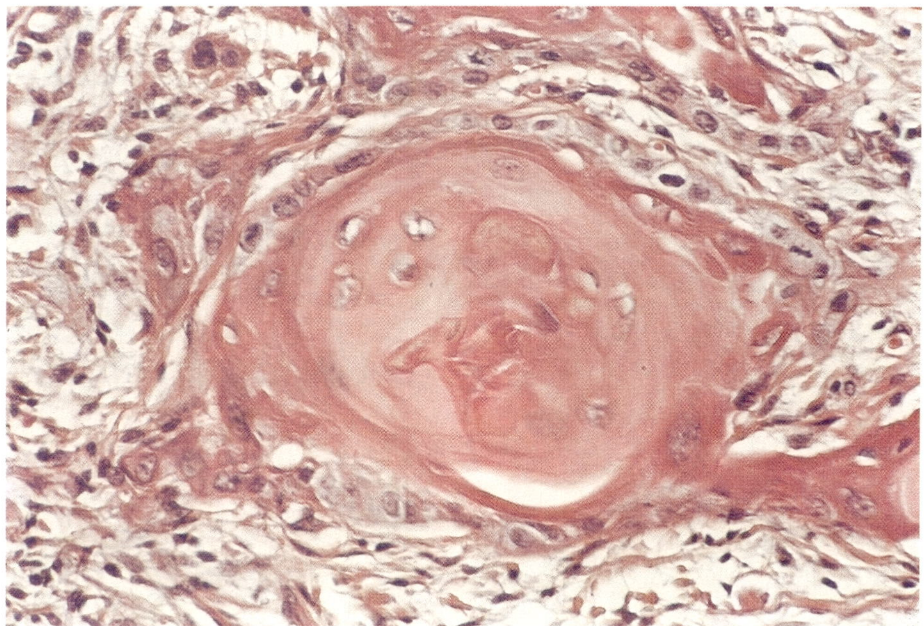
119

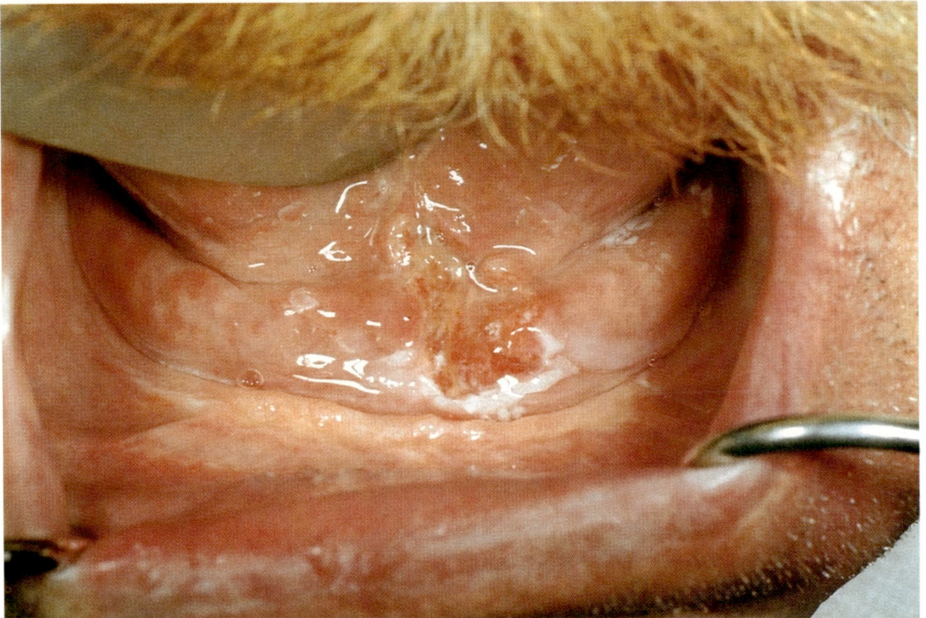

120

120 Shallow mucosal ulcer in the region of the anterior left floor of the mouth, showing a slight degree of marginal ridging and infiltration. Surrounding mucosa shows whitish discoloration. (Male aged 55; clinically, carcinoma suspected)

121 Largish groups of tumour cells showing marked cellular polymorphism and extensive signs of keratinisation.

122 High-power micrograph of tumour cells, showing an epithelial pearl.

Clinical management

Admission to hospital for fast-frozen section to confirm diagnosis histologically and immediate specific tumour therapy.

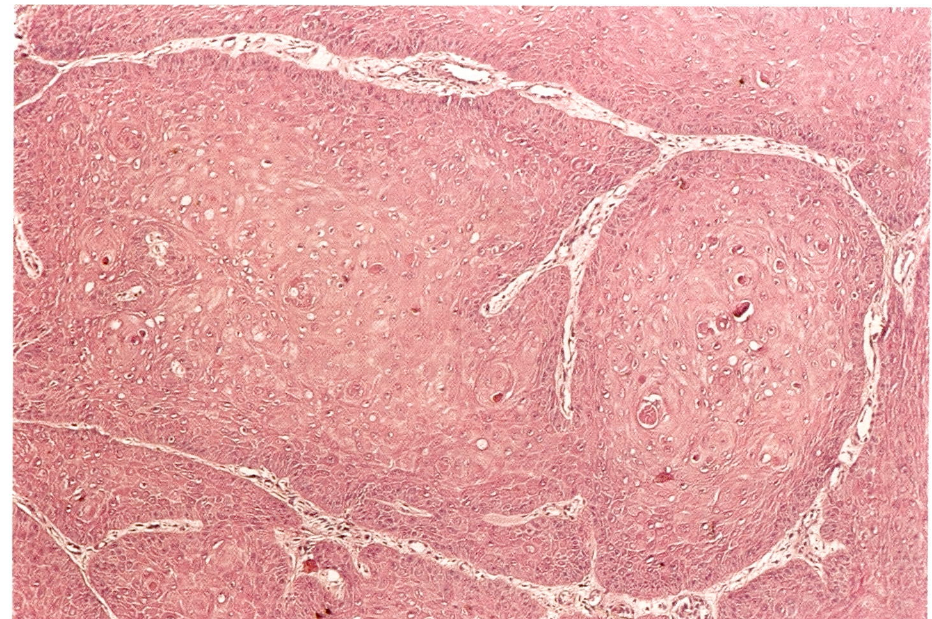

121

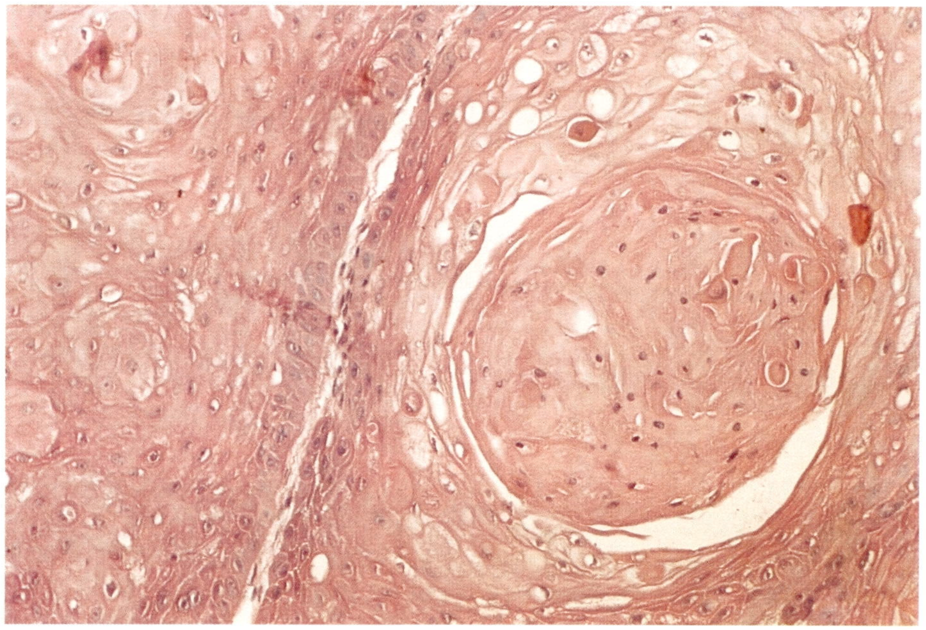

122

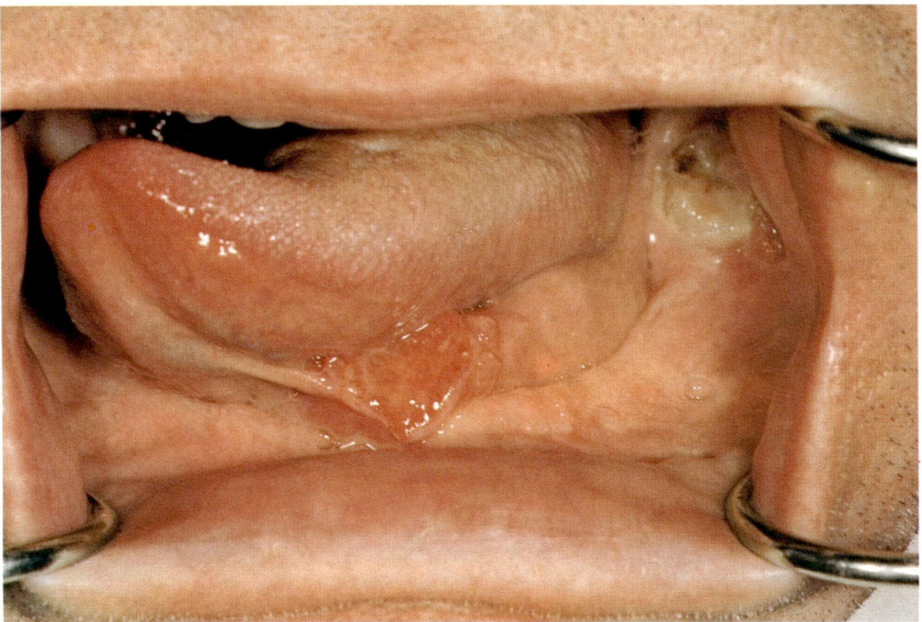

123

123 Bright red planar mucosal lesion, immediately sublingual, at the insertion of the frenum, 1 × 1cm in size, with induration in the surrounding area. (Male aged 63; clinically, malignancy suspected)

124 Groups of tumour cells showing a low degree of differentiation and considerable cellular and nuclear polymorphism. At the centre, an atypical mitotic figure can be seen. There are no signs of keratinisation.

125 Groups of tumour cells infiltrating the area of the vascular wall of a small arteriole.

126 Extensive tumour growth perineurally.

Clinical management

Admission to hospital for total excision of the lesion into healthy tissue and examination of fast-frozen section. In this case (Figures **123** to **125**) an early invasive carcinoma was found and specific tumour therapy initiated immediately.

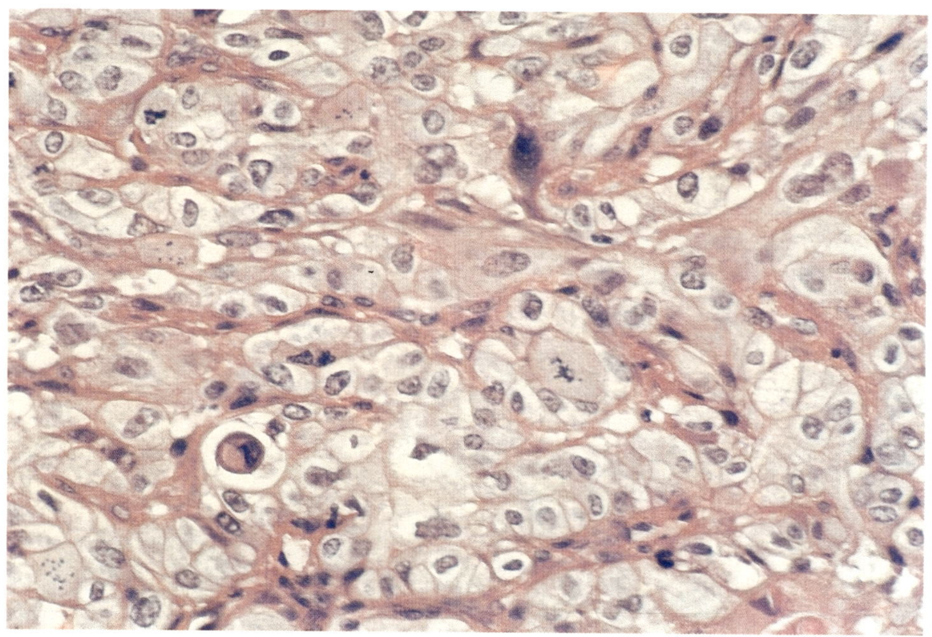

124

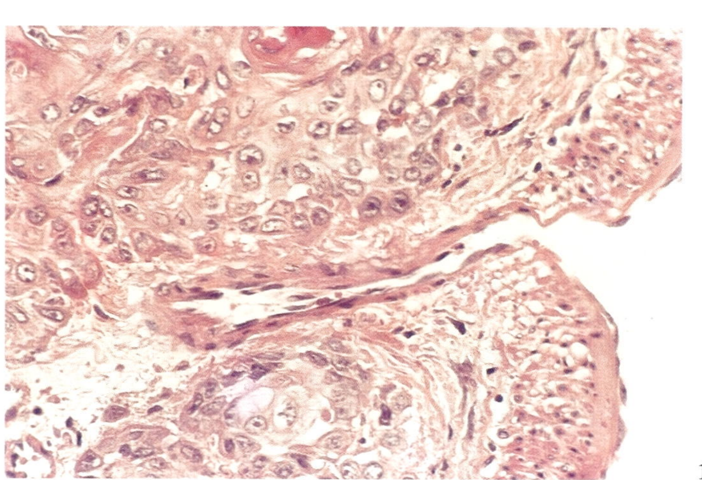

125

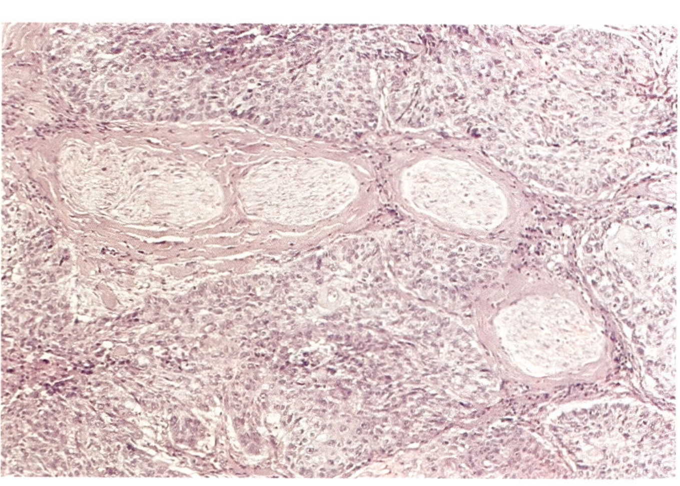

126

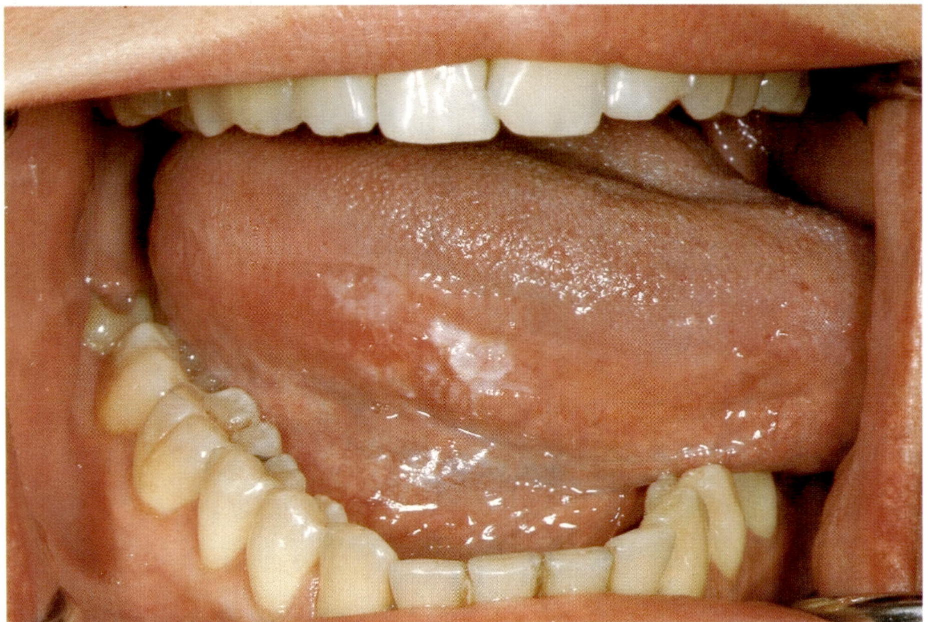

127

127 Extensive whitish changes in margin of the tongue, verrucous and slightly erosive, with some signs of infiltration. (Female aged 33; clinically, a precancerous lesion suspected)

128 Superficially, stratification of squamous epithelium is still maintained, with marked acanthosis. Basally, there is invasive growth of largish groups of atypical tumour cells. A dense inflammatory reaction can be seen in the stroma.

129 Tumour cone showing marked cellular and nuclear polymorphism and an epithelial pearl. In the surrounding area there is a dense inflammatory, predominantly lymphocytic, stroma reaction.

Clinical management

As the lesion is located in a high-risk area, admission to hospital is necessary for excision into healthy tissue and examination of a fast-frozen section. In this case (Figures **127** to **129**) an early invasive carcinoma was found and specific tumour therapy initiated immediately.

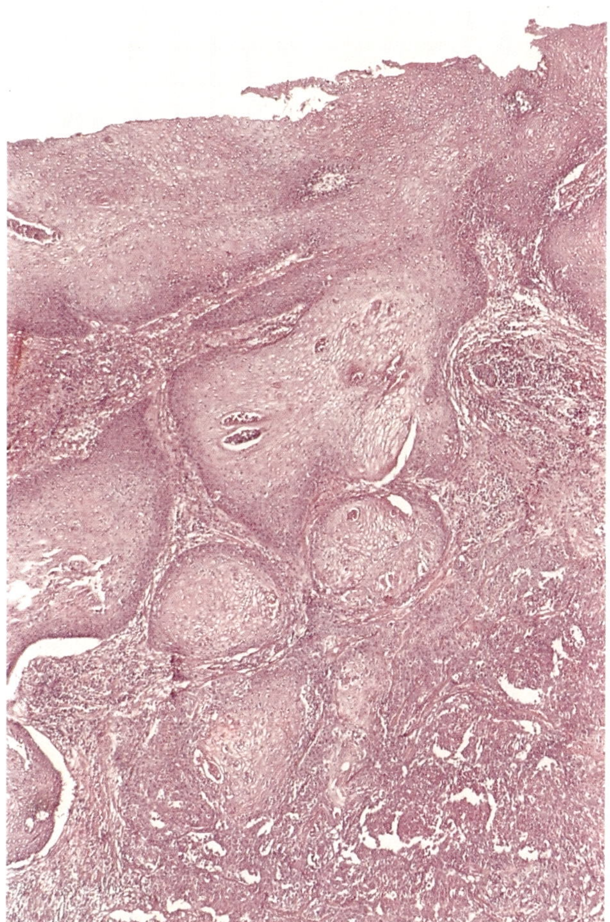

128

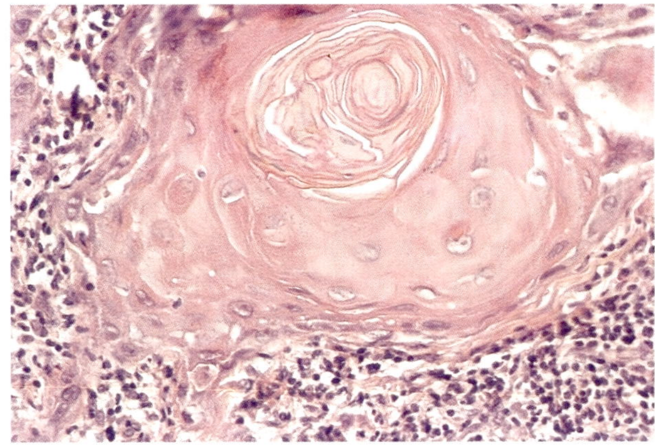

129

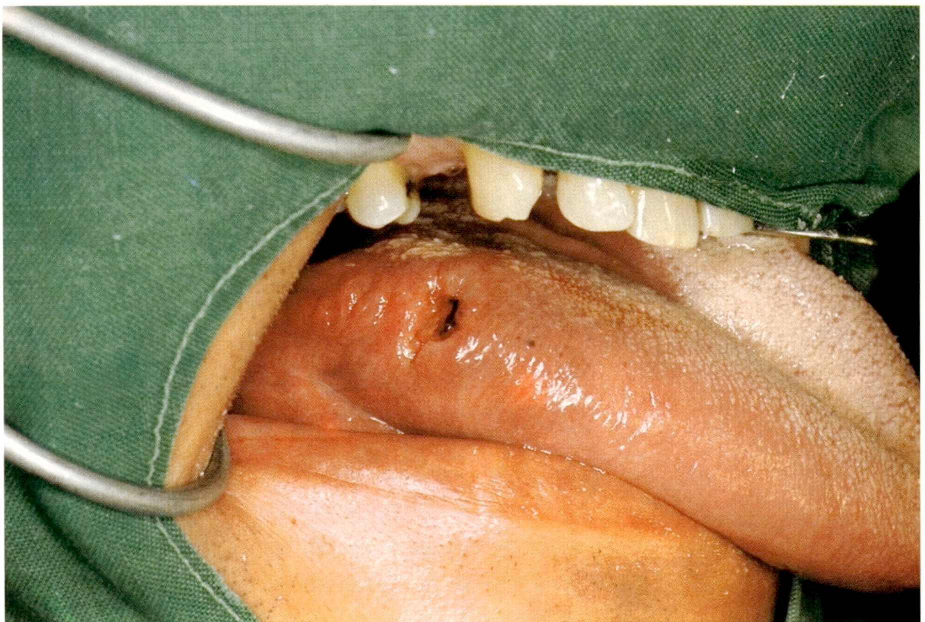

130

130 Deep ulceration, 1 × 1cm in size, with solid infiltration of surrounding area. (Male aged 52; clinically, carcinoma suspected)

131 Groups of clearly invasive tumour cells, with variable differentiation. On the left, basocellular differentiation with relatively uniform cell formations similar to basal cell carcinoma can be seen. To the right, spinocellular differentiation is evident, with marked cellular polymorphism and areas of keratinisation.

132 A large part of a tumour, with basocellular differentiation clearly in evidence.

133 Part of a tumour showing considerable cellular polymorphism and spinocellular differentiation.

Clinical management

Admission to hospital for examination of fast-frozen section to confirm diagnosis and immediate specific tumour therapy.

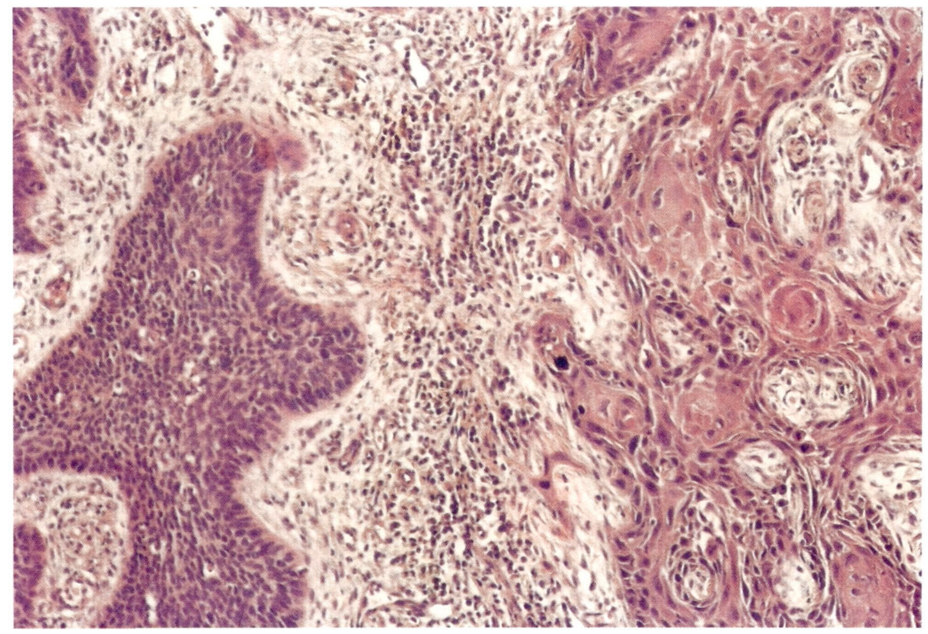

131

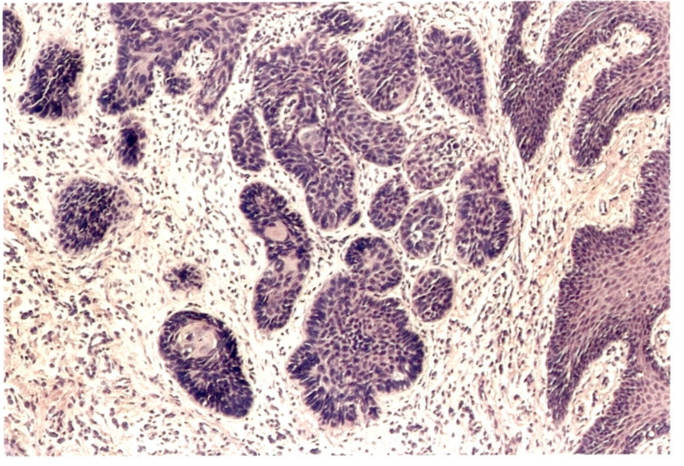

132

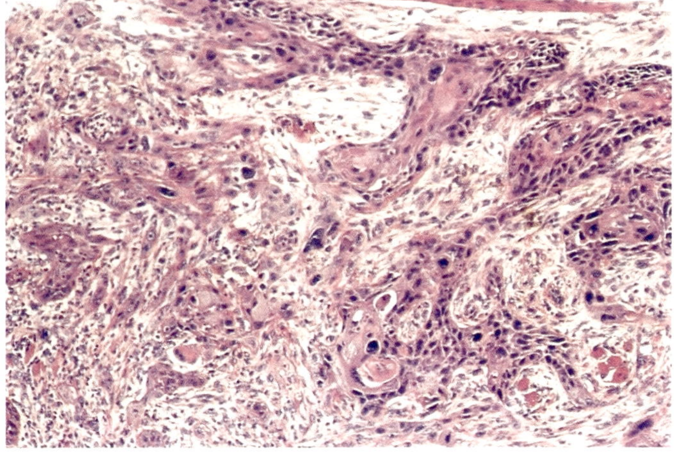

133

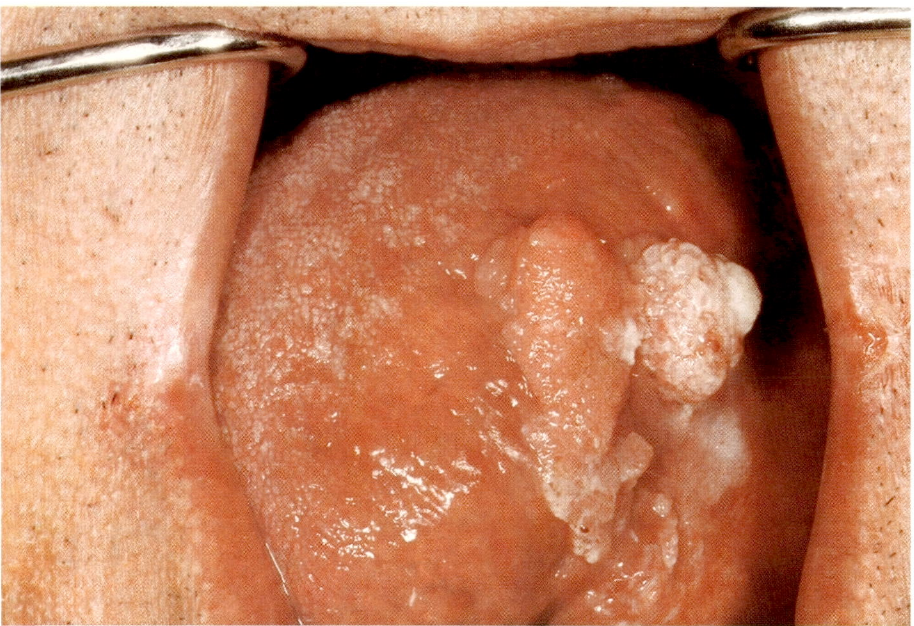

134

134 A verrucous, cauliflower-like hypertrophic lesion in the marginal mucosa of the tongue. The lesion is indurated and partly pedunculated, and shows whitish surface patches that cannot be rubbed off. (Male aged 65; clinically, carcinoma suspected)

135 Superficially and to the right, stratified epithelium is still maintained, with a slight degree of hyperparakeratosis. In the left half of the picture, gross invasive growth of groups of fusiform tumour cells can be seen.

136 In the upper part of the picture, stratified epithelium is still extant; inferior to this, are invasive irregular fusiform cell groups. There is a round cell reaction in the stroma.

137 High magnification of groups of tumour cells showing fusiform differentiation. The epithelial character of the tumour is not easily discernible in this area.

Clinical management

Admission to hospital for examination of fast-frozen section to verify diagnosis and immediate specific tumour therapy.

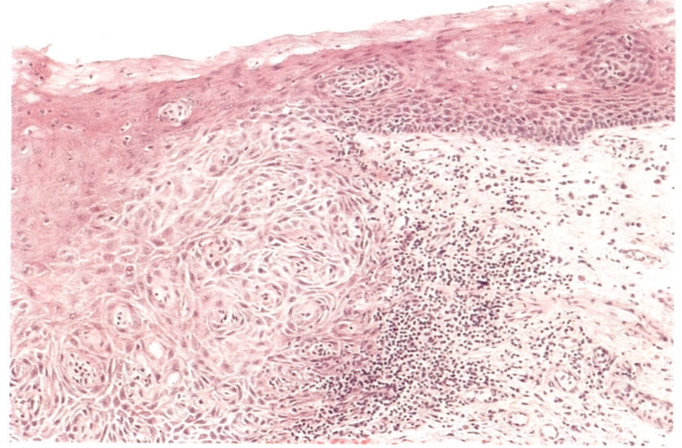
135

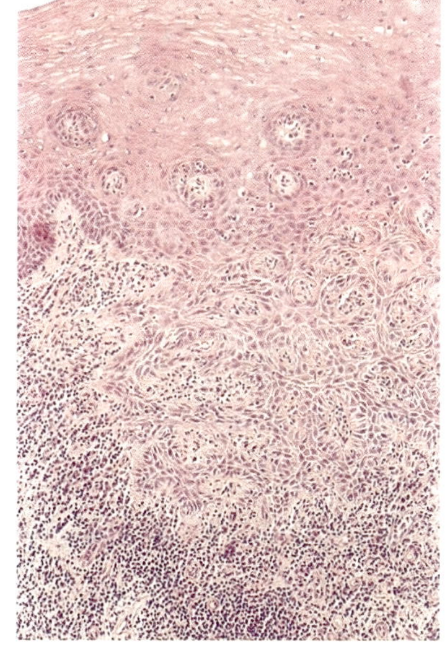
136

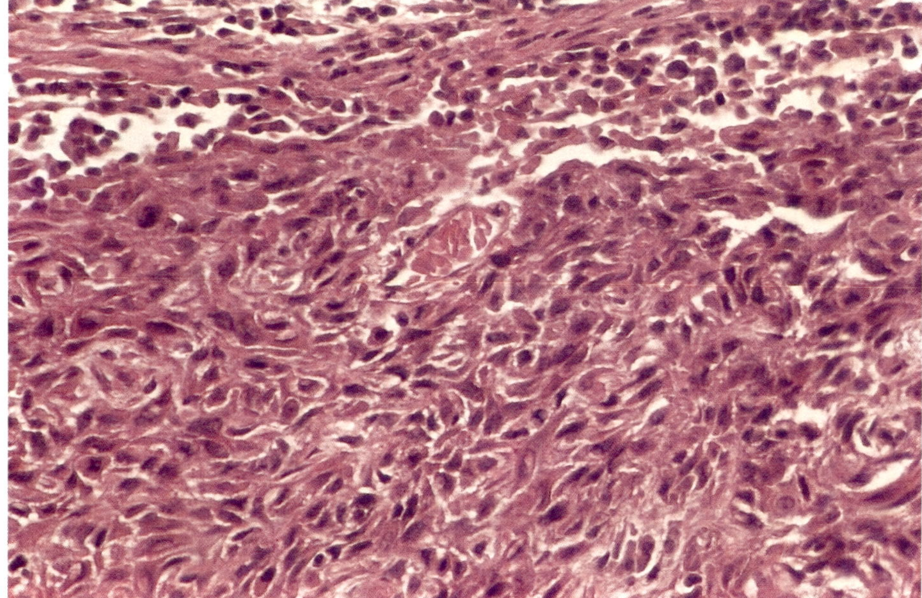
137

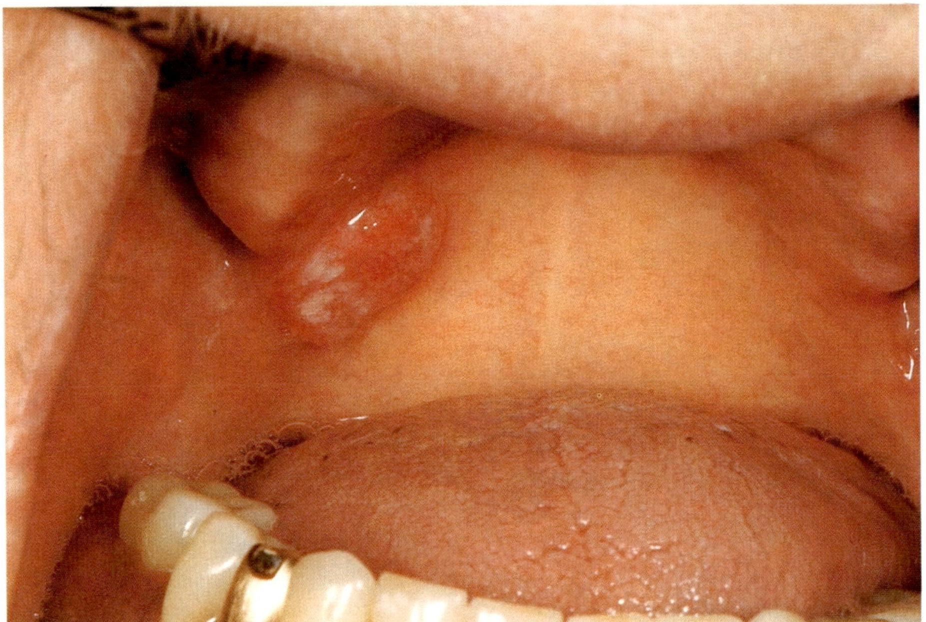

138

138 Immediately next to the right tuber, at the transition from hard to soft palate, is a large, dark-red hypertrophic mucosal lesion, 1 × 1cm in area; its surface shows erosion and whitish discoloration, and a downward and surrounding infiltration is clearly palpable. (Female aged 80; clinically, infiltration suggests carcinoma)

139 Atypical tumour cell groups show marked cellular and nuclear polymorphism. There are large areas of keratinisation, with transformation into keratin cysts.

140 Stratified keratin lamellae at the centre of the groups of tumour cells, demonstrated by special keratin staining. *(Chesa)*

Clinical management

Admission to hospital for examination of fast-frozen section to confirm diagnosis and immediate specific tumour therapy.

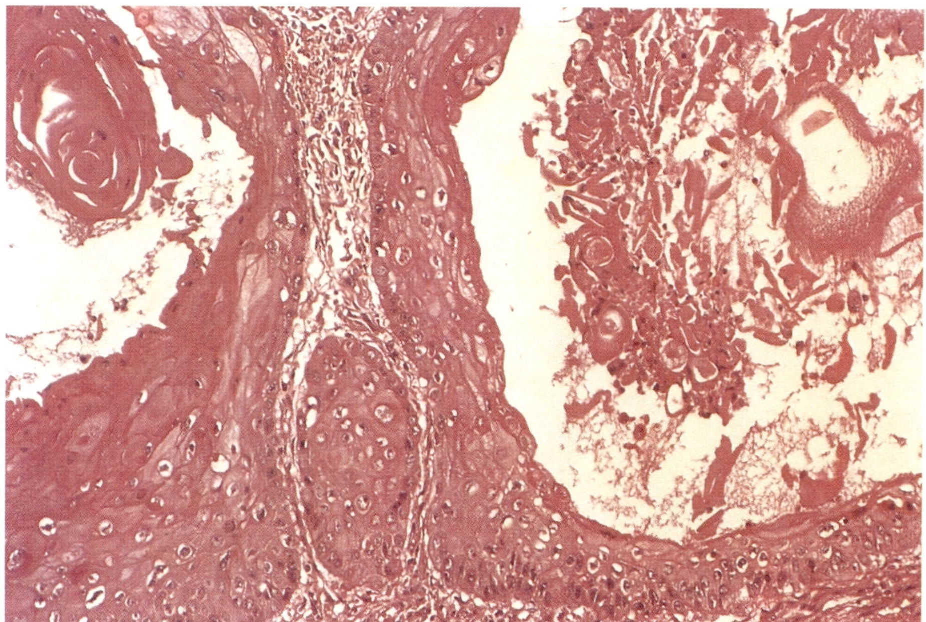
139

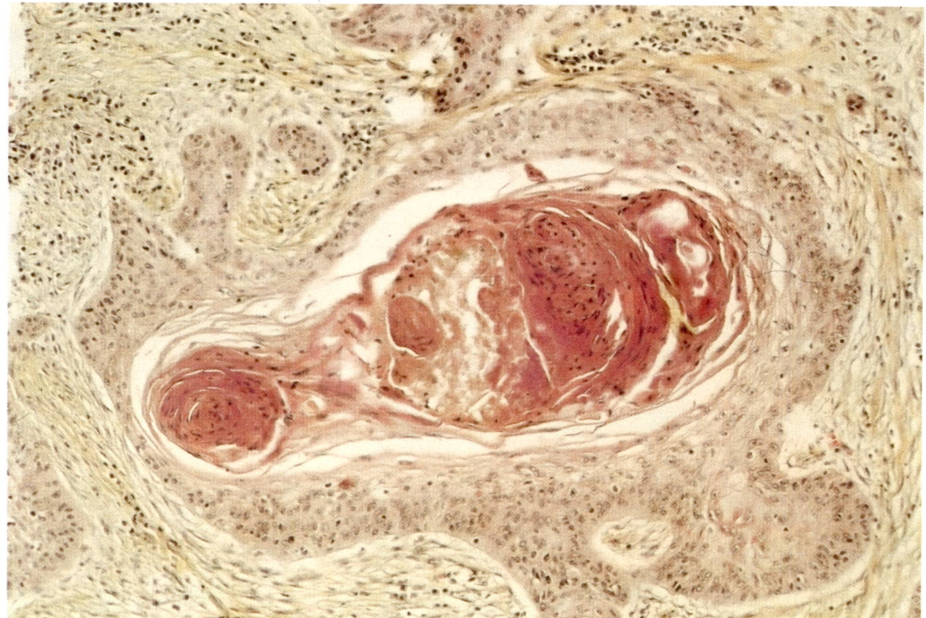
140

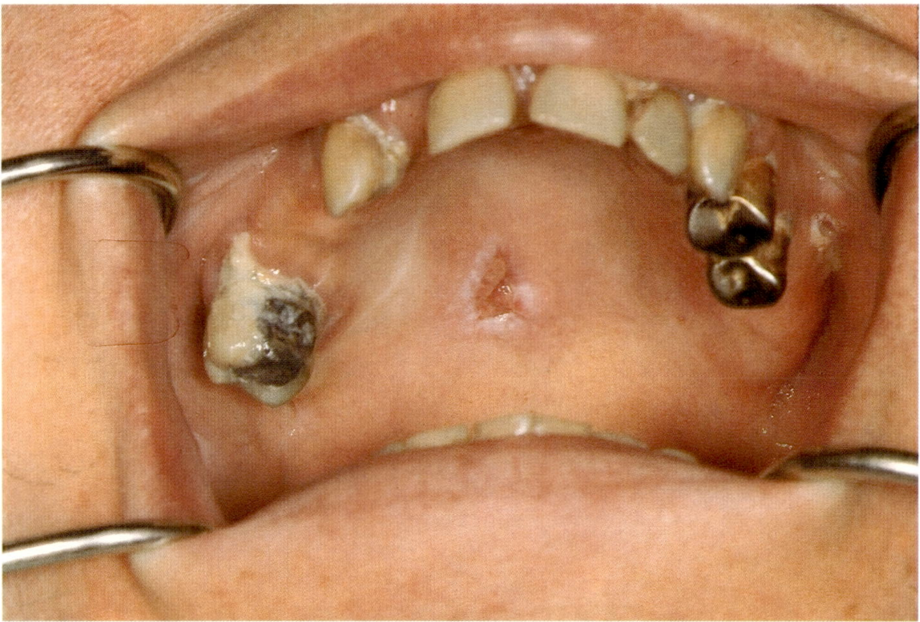

141

141 Ulceration at the posterior margin of the hard palate, immediately paramedial, 1 × 0.5cm in area, with marginal infiltration visible and palpable. Mucosal margins show whitish discoloration. (Female aged 65; clinically, malignancy suspected)

142 Highly polymorphic tumour cells showing definite nuclear hyperchromatism and polymorphism. Some areas show signs of keratinisation.

143 High magnification of tumour cell cone showing epidermoid stratification and marked cellular and nuclear polymorphism.

Clinical management

Admission to hospital for examination of fast-frozen section to verify diagnosis of carcinoma and immediate specific tumour therapy.

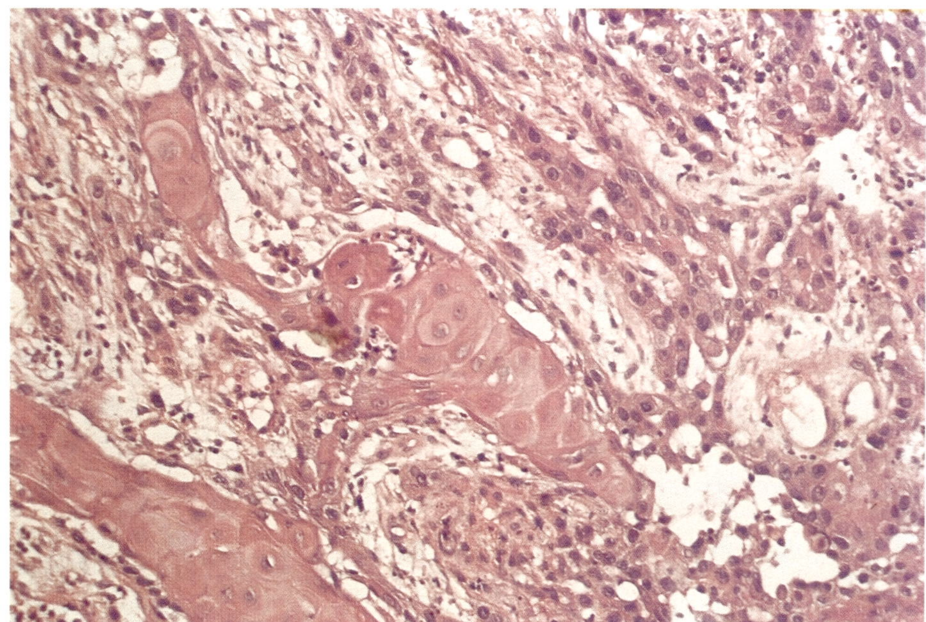

142

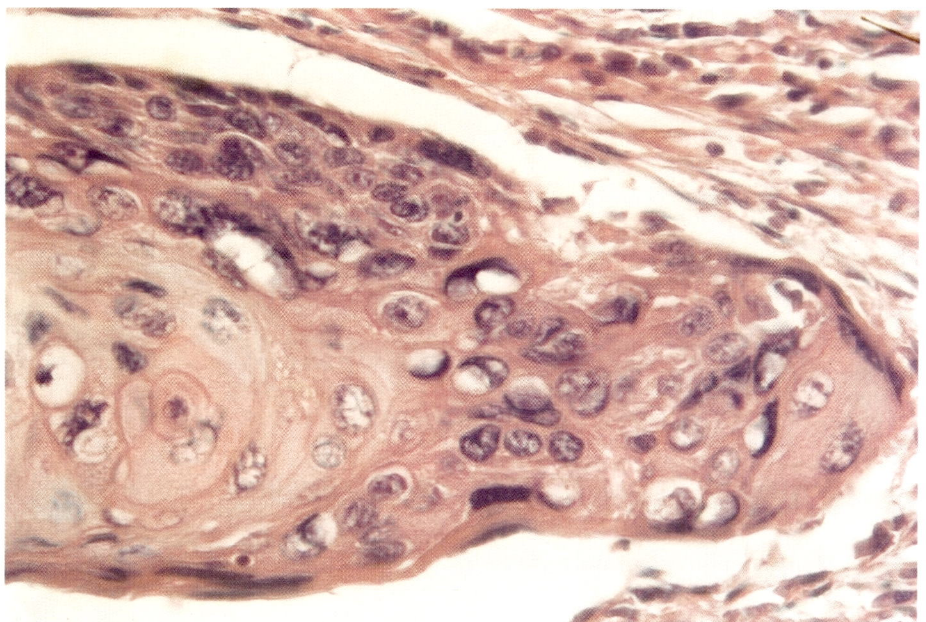

143

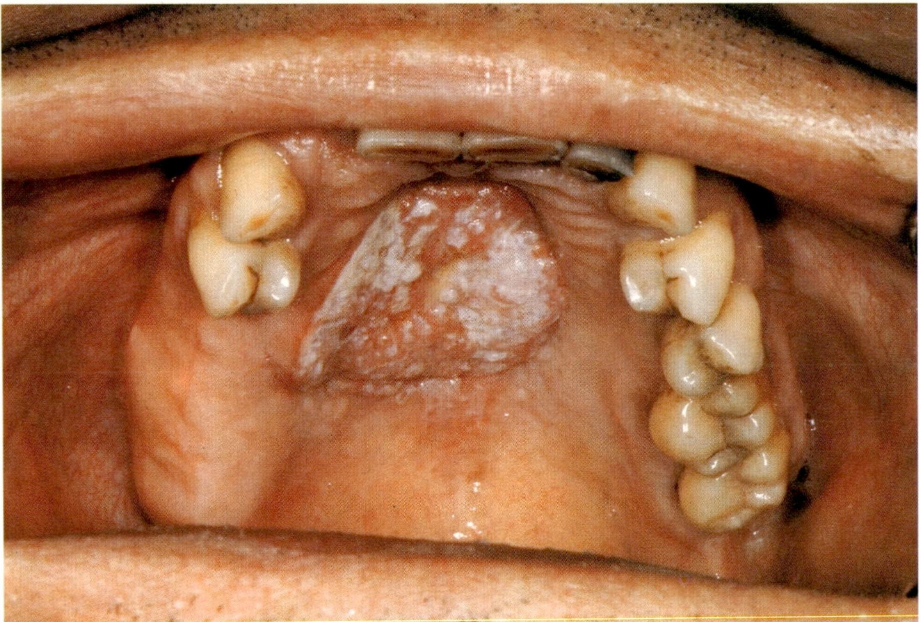

144

144 A clearly circumscribed lesion in palatal mucosa, 3.5 × 2.5cm in area, verrucous and erosive, with marked hypertrophy and a whitish nodular surface. Infiltration is not palpable beyond the raised margins. (Male aged 46; clinically, carcinoma suspected)

145 Narrow band of normal stratified epithelium, still extant (left). Adjacent to it, marked epithelial hyperplasia with both exophytic and endophytic components can be seen.

146 Detail from the centre of a deep-reaching endophytic cone showing the typical keratin plug at the centre. A dense inflammatory reaction in the stroma can also be seen.

147 Higher magnification of the tumour cone. Epithelial stratification is still discernible, but the basal cell layer is not definitely present. A moderate degree of cellular polymorphism is evident, and a wide keratin plug can be seen at the centre.

Clinical management

Admission to hospital for examination of fast-frozen section to confirm diagnosis and immediate specific tumour therapy. (Histologically this was a verrucous carcinoma, so radiotherapy and neck dissection were definitely not indicated.)

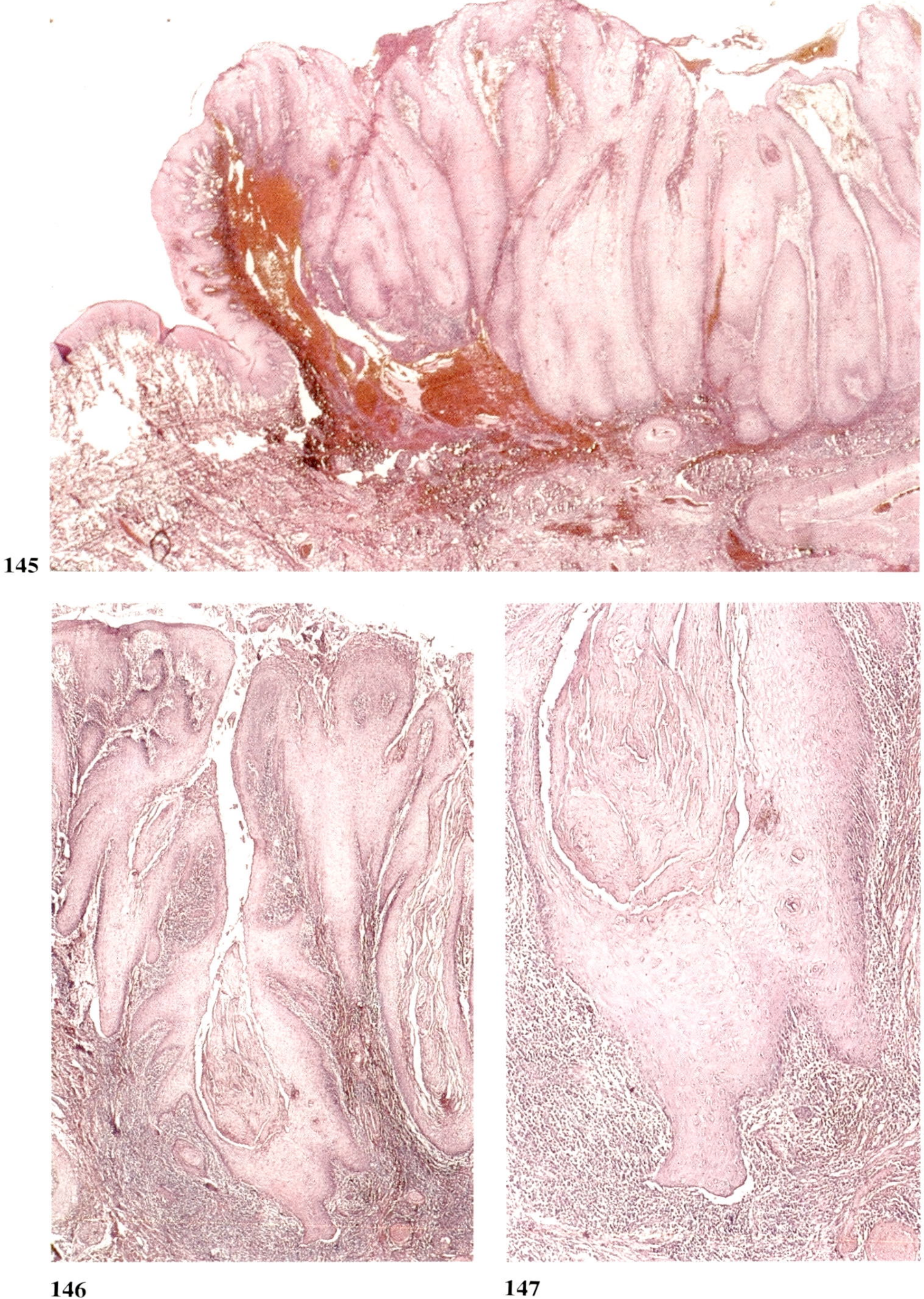

145

146

147

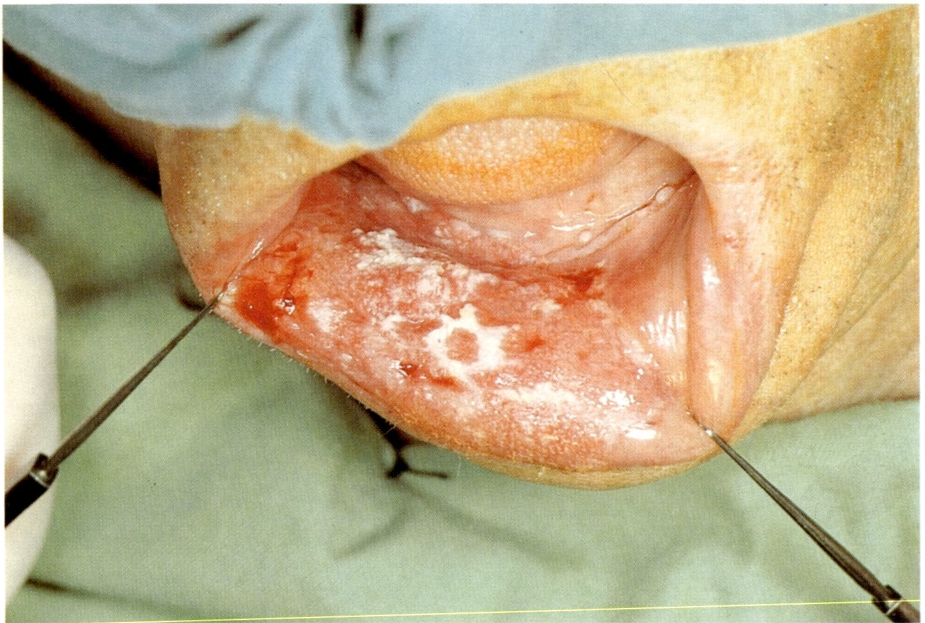

148

148 An extensive planar lesion, partly erosive, partly whitish and verrucous, in the mucosa of the lower lip, extending to the right buccal mucosa and lower alveolar process. The affected part and surrounding area are clearly indurated, and there is slight bleeding from the surface. (Male aged 74; clinically, precancerous lesion, at least, suspected)

149 The upper part of the micrograph shows the basal part of extant epithelium, with a high degree of dysplasia. Inferior to this, is a broad-based invasion of tumour cell groups and areas of keratinisation. There is a lymphocytic reaction in the stroma.

150 Detail from a tumour cone, with keratinisation of numerous individual cells (dyskeratosis).

Clinical management

Admission to hospital for excision of the lesion into healthy tissue and examination of fast-frozen section. In this case (Figures **148** to **150**), a carcinoma was found and more radical surgery and follow-up cancer therapy were initiated.

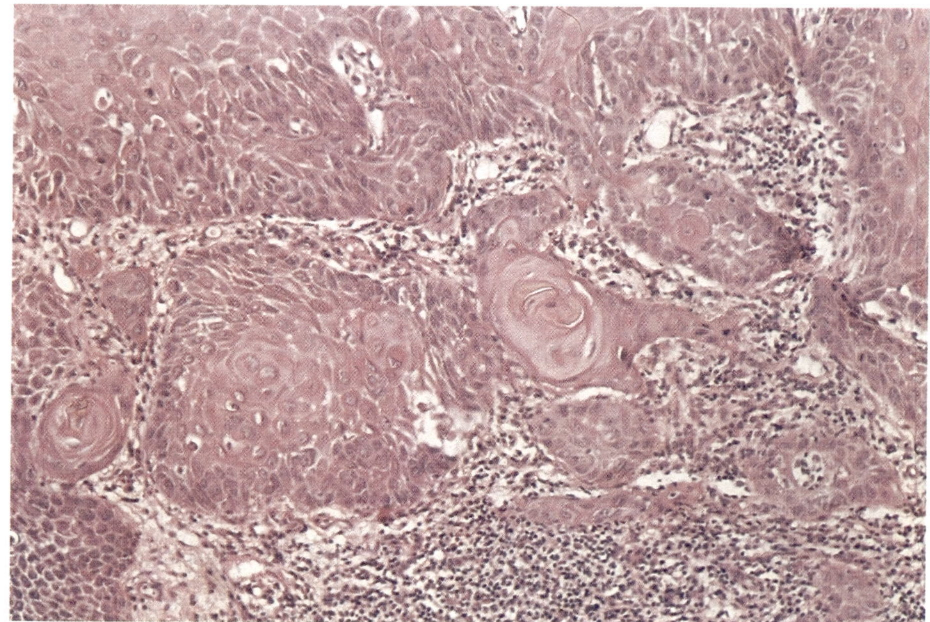
149

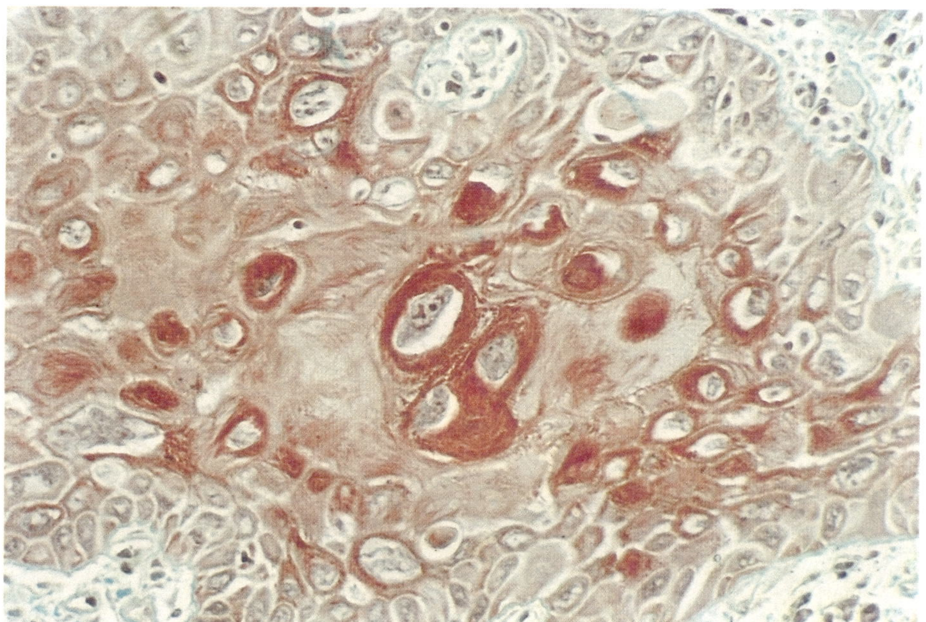
150

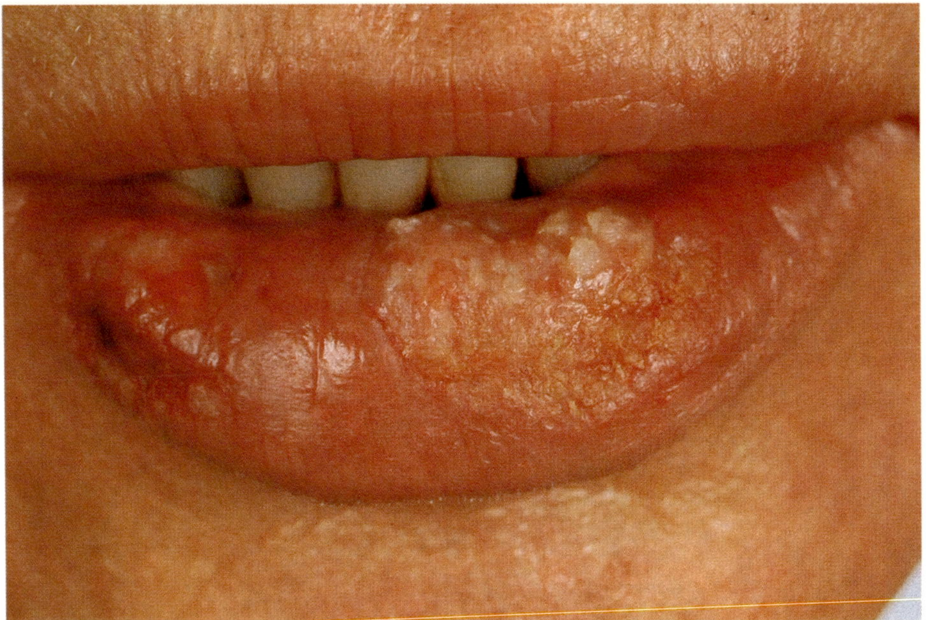

151

151 Verrucous, partly erosive mucosal lesion showing whitish-yellow discoloration in the region of the lower lip-red, 2 × 1cm in area. Towards the edges and deeper down, infiltration is clearly palpable. (Male aged 65; clinically, carcinoma suspected)

152 Superficially, stratified epithelium is partly maintained with marked hyperorthokeratosis. Groups of tumour cells in the stroma beneath are clearly invasive and a dense inflammatory stroma reaction is evident.

153 Detail from an invasive tumour cone showing considerable cellular and nuclear polymorphism, with keratinisation of numerous individual cells.

Clinical management

Admission to hospital for biopsy and examination of fast-frozen section to confirm diagnosis. If confirmed surgical removal should be completed, and follow-up cancer therapy instituted.

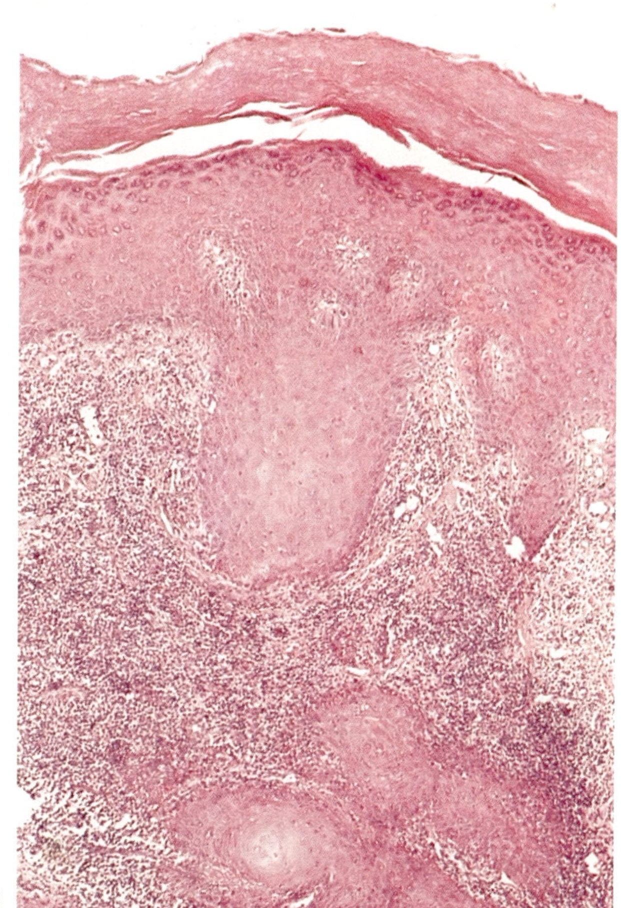

152

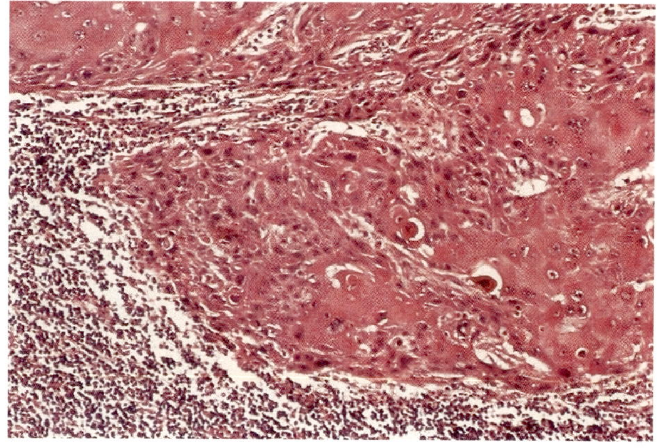

153

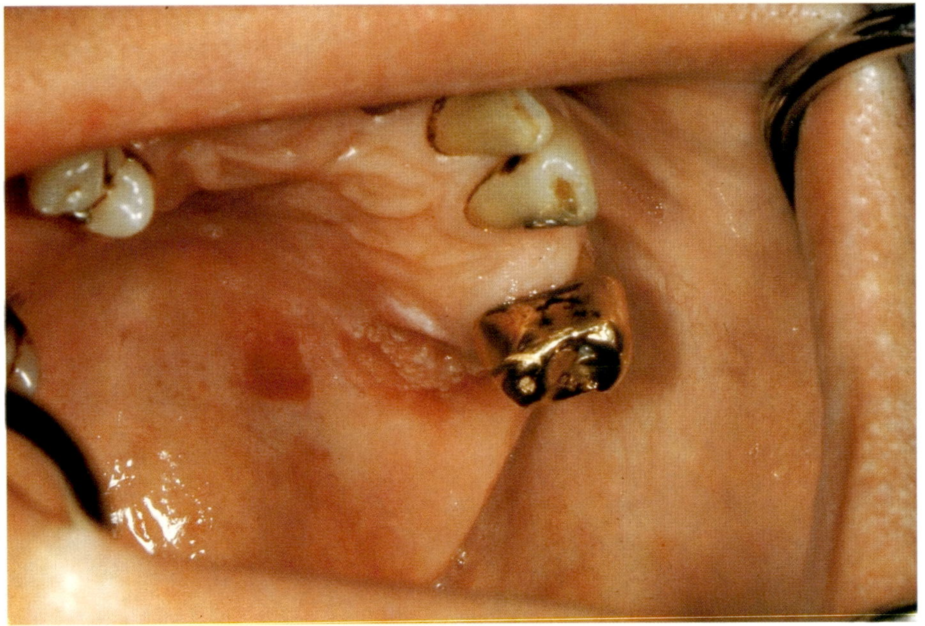

154

154 Ulceration, 1 × 1cm in area, with raised margins showing whitish discoloration, palatinal to 1st upper premolar on the left, with no direct connection to periodontium of the tooth. (Male aged 56; clinically, carcinoma suspected)

155 Groups of tumour cells with predominantly fusiform differentiation. Occasional signs of a tendency to keratinise are also in evidence.

156 High-power micrograph of detail, showing small area of keratinisation in the midst of tumour cells with fusiform differentiation. There is marked cellular and nuclear polymorphism.

Clinical management

Admission to hospital for examination of fast-frozen section to confirm diagnosis and immediate specific tumour therapy.

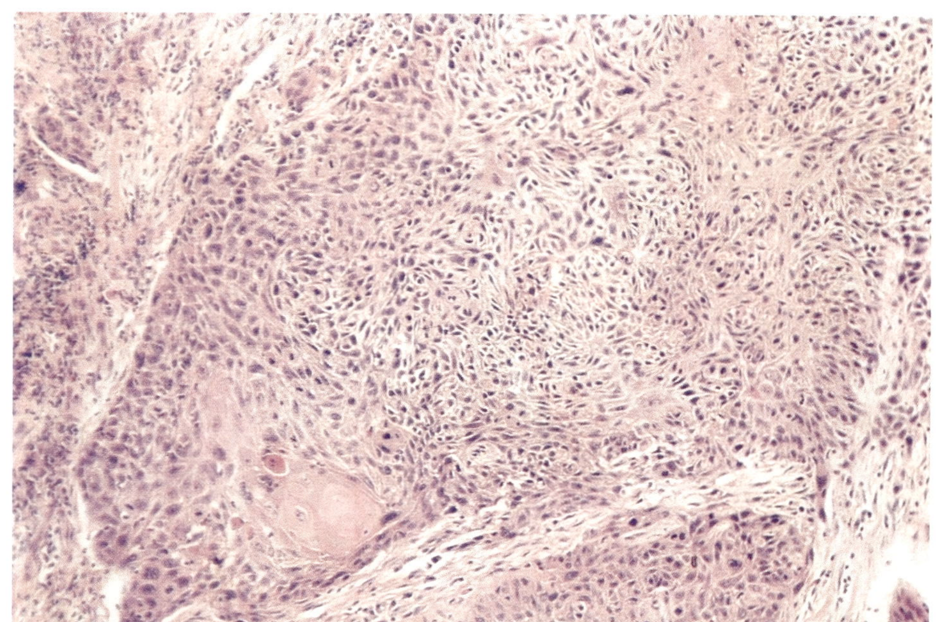
155

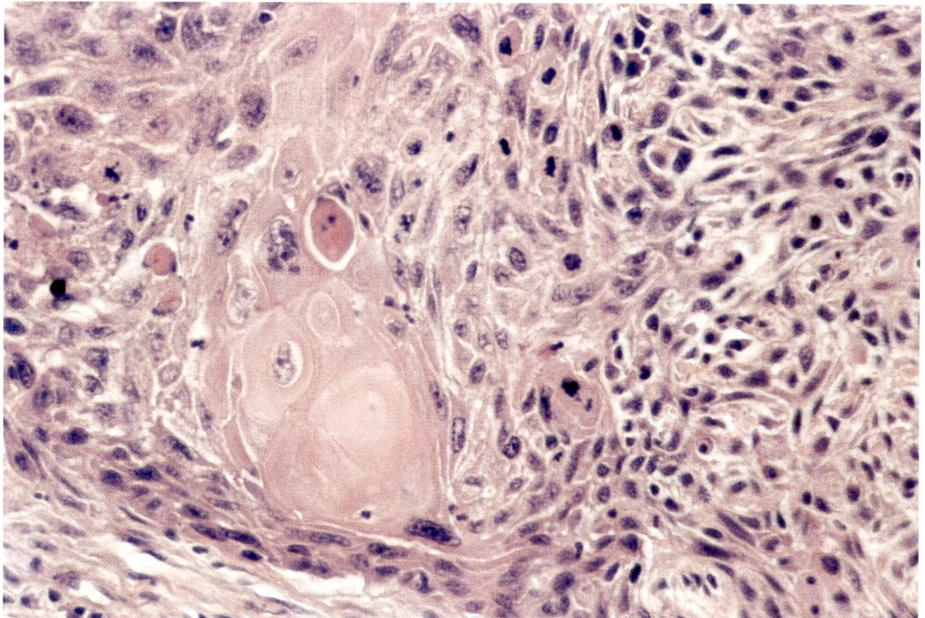
156

5 Differential diagnosis

The diagnosis of leukoplakias requiring treatment is based on a process of elimination. A number of established syndromes must be considered in the clinical assessment and eliminated, where appropriate, by histological examination. Syndromes of this type include local anomalies or diseases, but they are generally oral manifestations of dermatological conditions (Table 12). When such conditions involve the oral cavity only, and are not in evidence in the external skin, their diagnosis may prove difficult.

Table 12 Major Syndromes to be Distinguished from Oral Leukoplakia by Differential Diagnosis

Local anomalies or conditions	Dermatological conditions
White sponge naevus	Lichen planus
Smoker's palate	Discoid lupus erythematosus
Viral focal epithelial hyperplasias	Erythema multiforme
Glossitis migrans	Pemphigus vulgaris
Glossitis rhombica mediana	Psoriasis

A number of inflammatory conditions affecting the oral mucosa may also present as whitish changes and thus make diagnosis difficult for the inexperienced. Some of these changes may also carry a risk of malignant degeneration after persisting for some time, but they are not precancerous lesions in themselves. In general, they should be regarded as additional irritant factors in carcinogenesis and accordingly as risk-factors. Conditions of this type include discoid lupus erythematosus, submucous fibrosis (a condition seen mainly in India), lichen planus and the glossitis forming part of the tertiary syphilis syndrome.

Nonspecific ulceration of the mucosa needs to be differentiated from ulcerative forms of early cancer. Any ulcer that refuses to heal must be suspected of being malignant. In cases of doubt, histological examination is essential and is indicated when conservative therapy has proved ineffective for a period of 10 days at most.

White sponge naevus (naevus spongiosus albus mucosae)

This malformation of the mucosa is not easy to distinguish from symptomatic leukoplakias. It normally occurs early, as a congenital and familial lesion, and increases during later life. Macroscopic inspection shows a spongy, plicated mucosa with greyish-white discoloration. The cheek is the preferred site, while the tongue or other areas of the oral mucosa are less frequently affected. Histologically, the condition is harmless and there is no dysplasia.

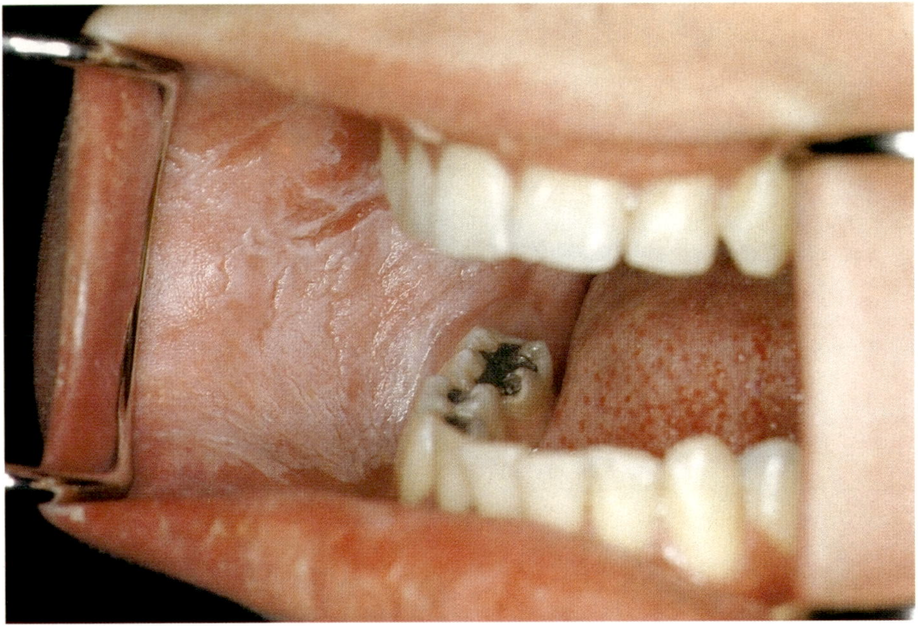

157

157 Homogeneous greyish-white discoloration of the mucosa of the whole cheek, which is slightly hypertrophic, doughy and plicated. (Male aged 17, healthy; clinically non-suspect)

158 Planar stratified epithelium with marked acanthosis and hyperparakeratosis, well developed rete pegs and a minor degree of subepithelial fibrosis.

159 Enlarged detail of epithelial ridges showing normal epithelial differentiation and no basal cell hyperplasia.

160 Superficial epithelium showing parakeratosis and oedematous cells.

Clinical management

Eliminate risk-factors, inform and instruct the patient. Follow-up as part of general treatment measures at long intervals. No treatment is required.

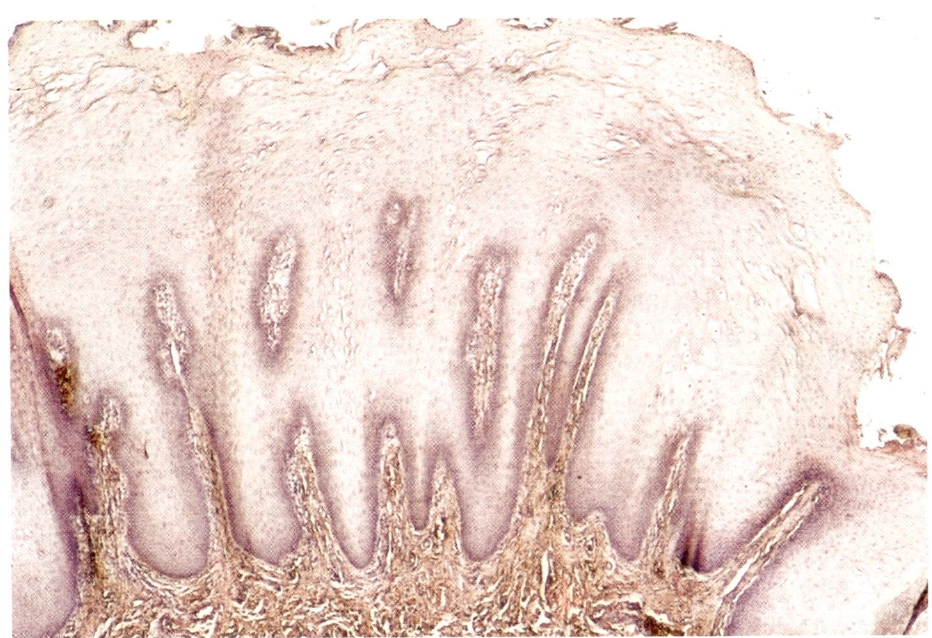

158

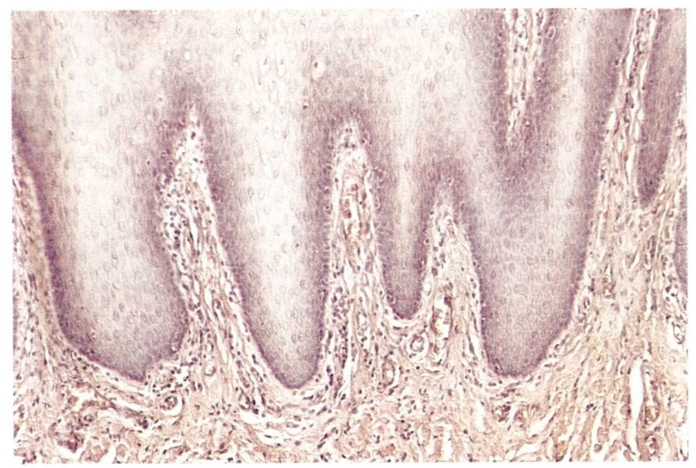

159

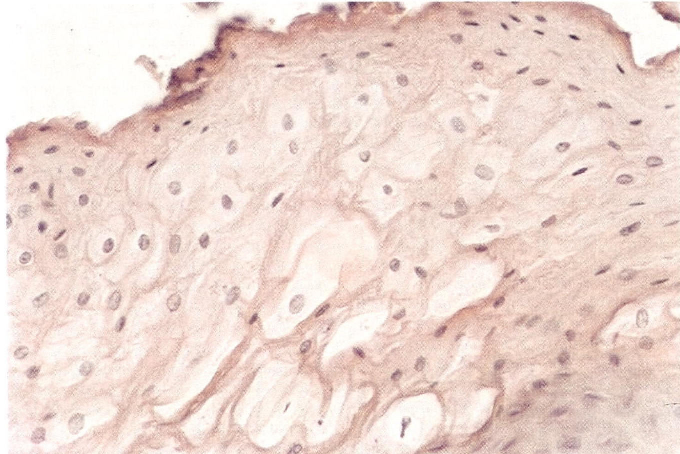

160

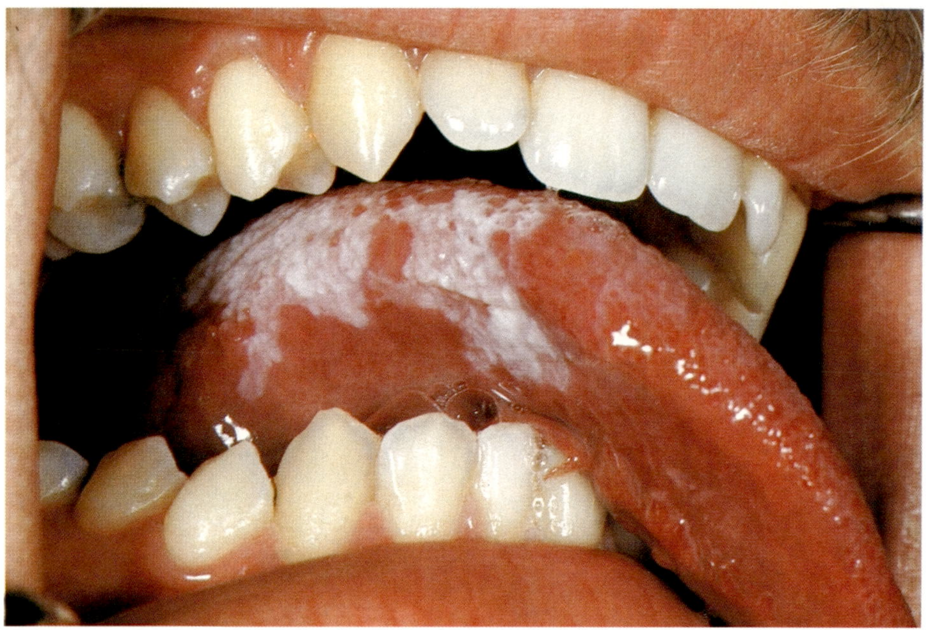

161

161 In the lateral margin of the tongue is a whitish, well defined change that shows a slight degree of plication and cannot be rubbed off. There is no ulceration or infiltration, and the patch is doughy to furry in consistency. (Male aged 18, healthy; clinically non-suspect)

162 Normal stratification of epithelium with well defined rete pegs, marked acanthosis and hyperparakeratosis. Cell bodies are spongy and oedematous.

163 Prickle cell layer with demonstrable intracellular glycogen. *(PAS)*

164 High-power micrograph of basal epithelium. Basal cells show normal relations, prickle cells are normal, nuclei are regular; there is nothing to indicate dysplasia.

Clinical management

As the margin of the tongue is a high-risk location, biopsy was taken as a safety measure to exclude dysplasia. In this case (Figures **161** to **164**), no dysplasia was found. Eliminate risk-factors, inform and instruct the patient, and follow-up as part of general treatment measures, at long intervals. No treatment is required.

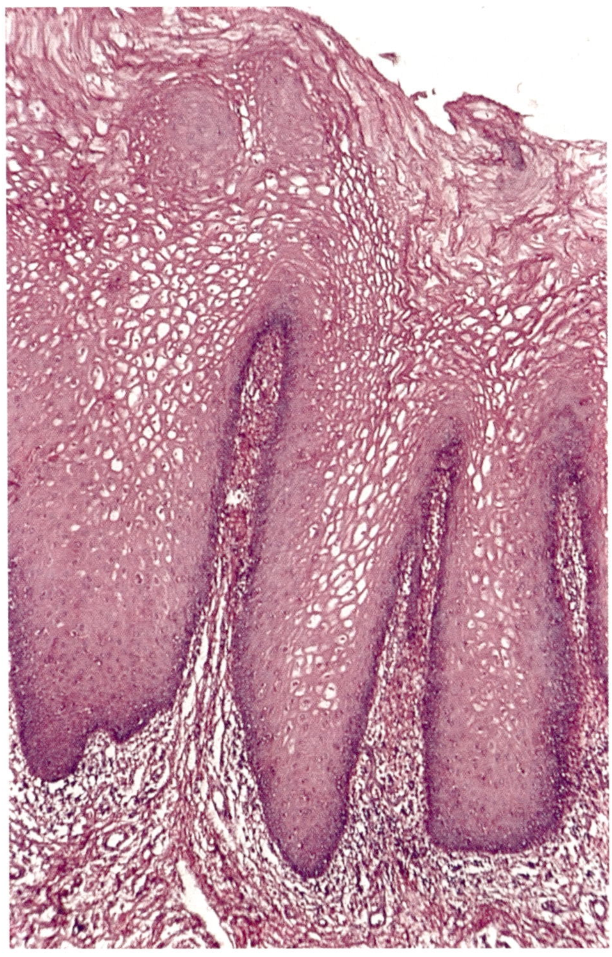

162

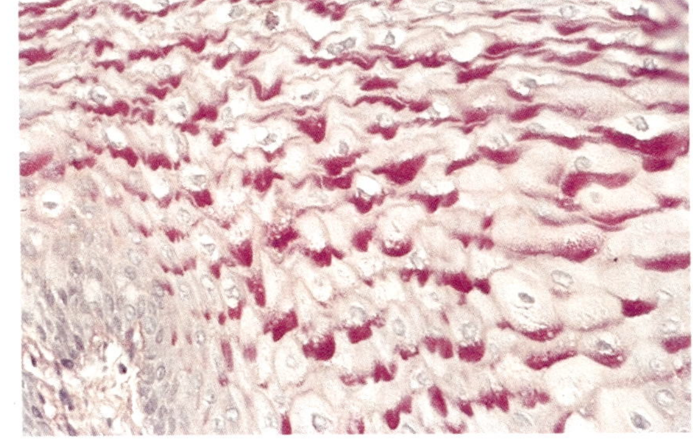

163

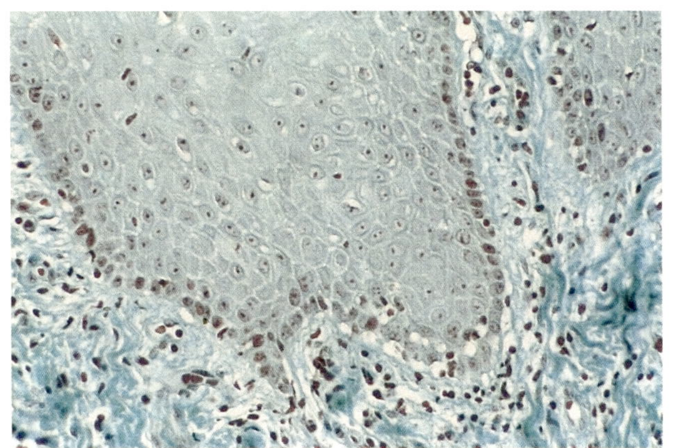

164

Smoker's palate (leukokeratosis nicotinica palati)

This special form of leukokeratosis is found in the region of transition from hard to soft palate. It has the additional characteristic of multiple inflamed orifices of mucous gland ducts appearing in the form of red spots. This condition is seen chiefly in pipe smokers and in people who habitually take very hot food and drink. The temperature of the food appears to play a major role in the pathogenesis. It is stated that smoker's palate almost never shows malignant degeneration and therefore does not rank as a precancerous condition.

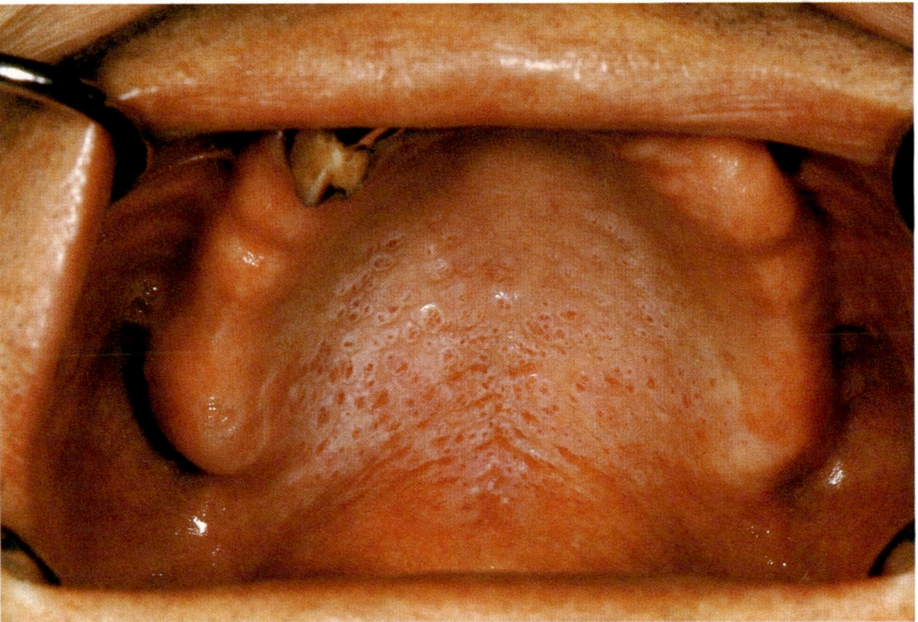

165

165 Diffuse, faintly greyish-white discoloration of the whole mucosa in the posterior part of the hard palate and transition to soft palate. Swelling is clearly visible at the orifices of accessory salivary glands, which appear red. (Male aged 74, heavy smoker; clinically non-suspect)

166 Epithelium showing focal acanthosis and increased numbers of basal rete pegs. To the right, is a glandular duct with squamous epithelium showing metaplasia. There is a dense inflammatory stroma reaction.

167 Rete pegs clearly lengthened and anastomosing, with some signs of keratinising tendency indicating slightly abnormal epithelial differentiation. There is inflammatory infiltration of connective tissue.

168 Squamous metaplasia of the epithelium in a fairly large glandular duct, but no epithelial dysplasia.

Clinical management

Eliminate risk-factors (no smoking). No treatment is required.

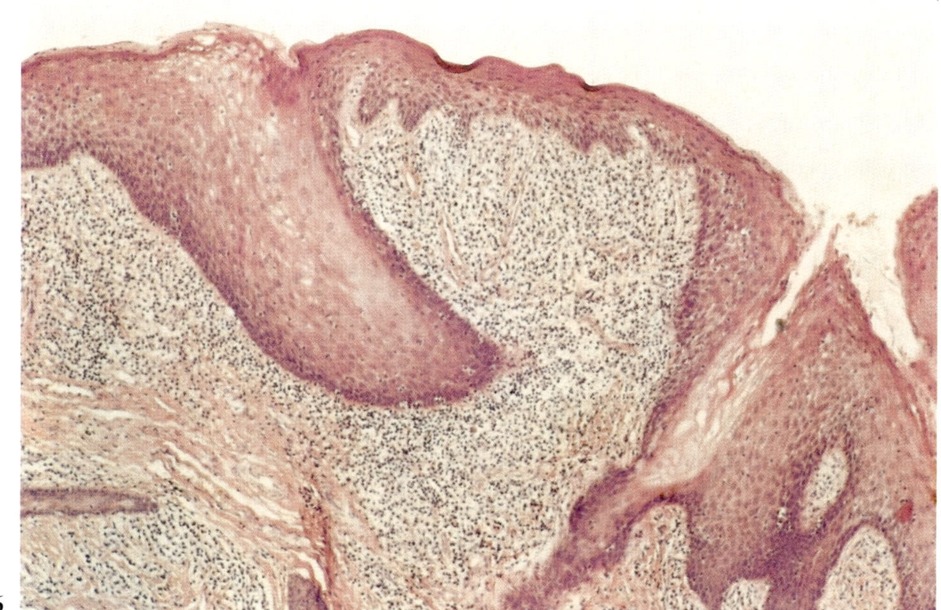
166

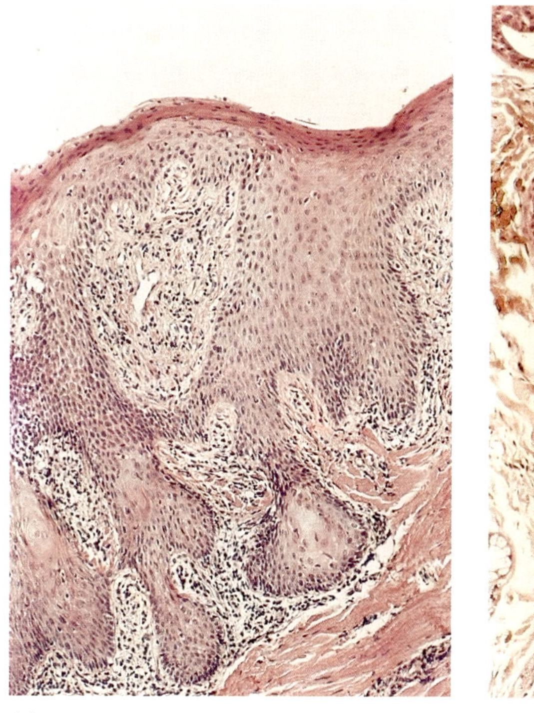
167

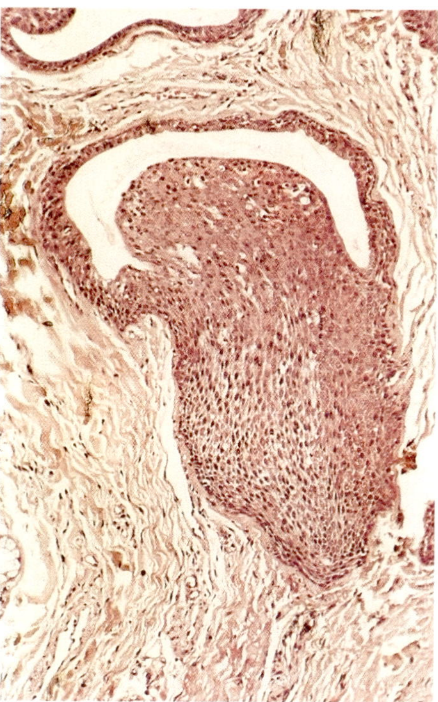
168

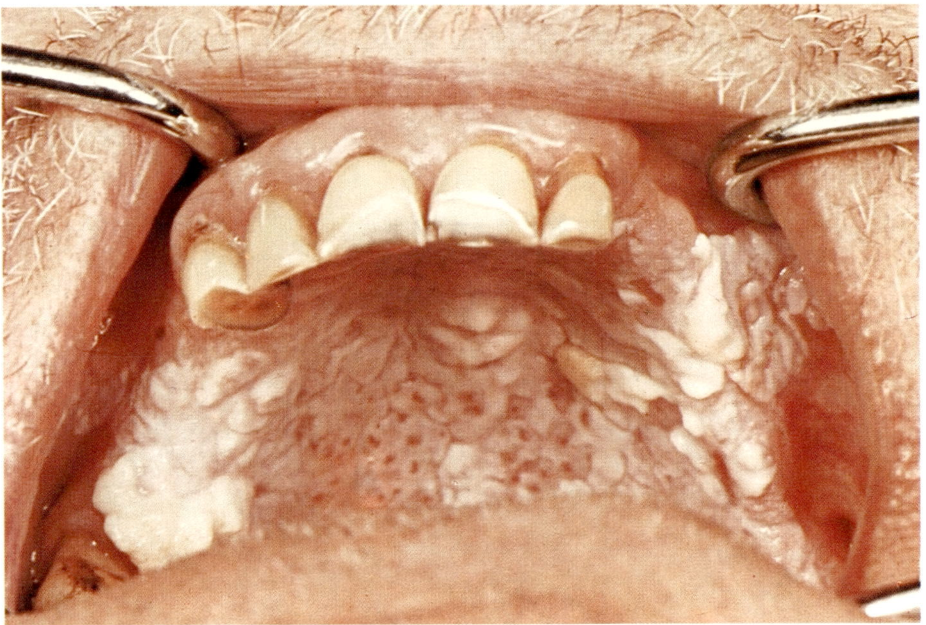

169

169 A thick, hard, whitish lesion in the region of the upper alveolar process, and bands of whitish discoloration of palatal mucosa with prominent efferent ducts of accessory salivary glands. (Male aged 70, heavy smoker; clinically, malignancy suspected in region of alveolar processes)

170 Duct of small salivary gland of the palate with squamous metaplasia of duct-epithelium and ulceration of the surface epithelium.

171 Efferent duct of a small palatal salivary gland showing marked squamous metaplasia of the epithelium. The lumen contains thickened secretion and desquamated epithelial cells.

172 Papillomatous exophytic epithelium with acanthosis and a narrow area of orthokeratosis. Basal parts show occasional disorganised rete peg formations. Inflammatory infiltration of stroma is evident.

173 Basal epithelial rete pegs at high magnification. The basal cell layer is not clearly definable, and cells show a low degree of nuclear polymorphism. In addition, there are increased numbers of mitotic figures, limited to the basal and suprabasal areas. No atypical mitotic figures can be seen.

Clinical management

Admission to hospital for biopsies from several areas of leukoplakia that appeared suspicious, and examination of fast-frozen sections. In this case (Figures **169** to **173**) no carcinoma was found. Histological examination showed a moderate degree of dysplasia. Follow-up observation should be undertaken every four to eight weeks, and the patient advised to stop smoking.

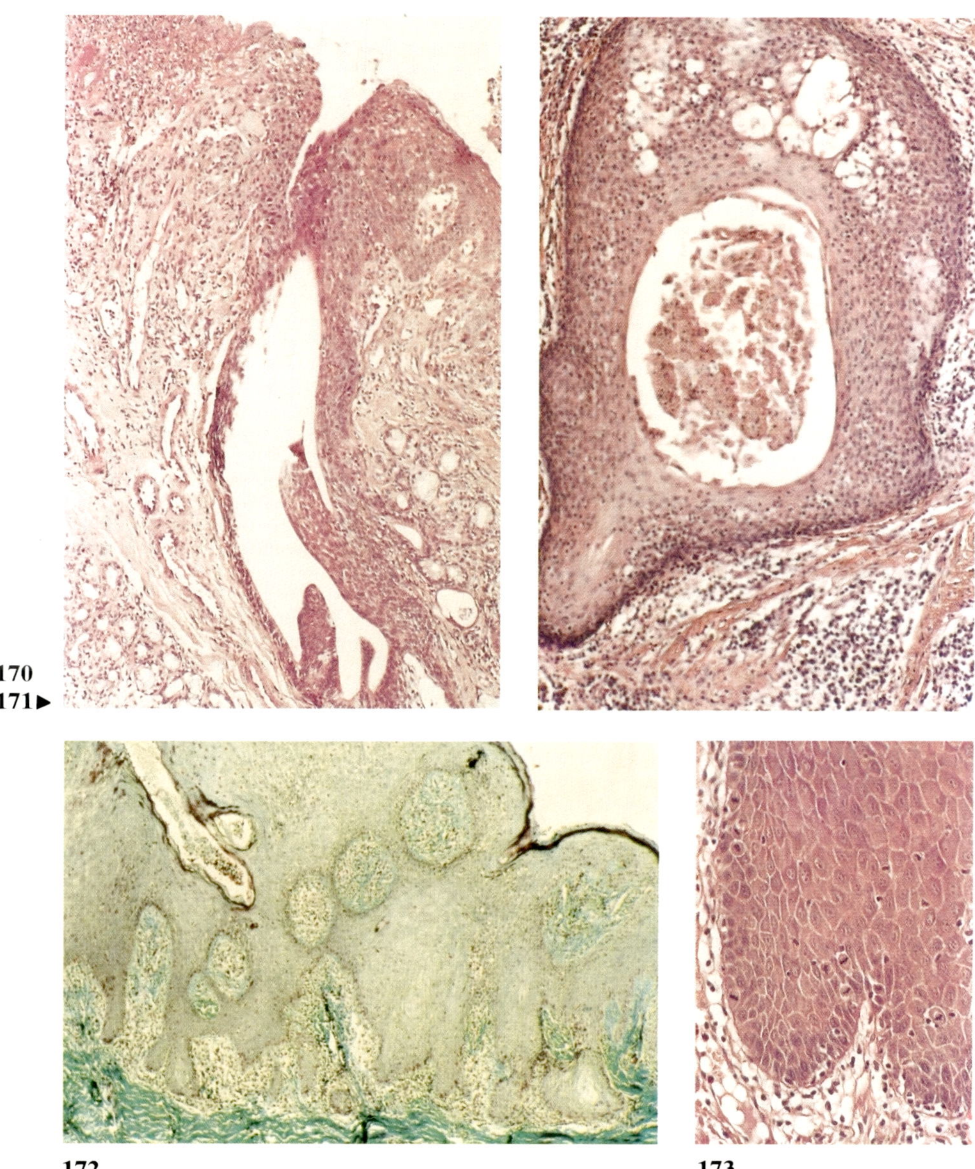

170
171▶

172

173

Geographic tongue (lingua geographica, glossitis migrans)

Geographic tongue is a condition of unknown aetiology occurring in relatively young adults. It is characterised by fairly large, reddish patches on the dorsum of the tongue, often with whitish margins, that may change their shape (migration). The condition is harmless and does not require treatment. Spontaneous remission for no apparent reason is common.

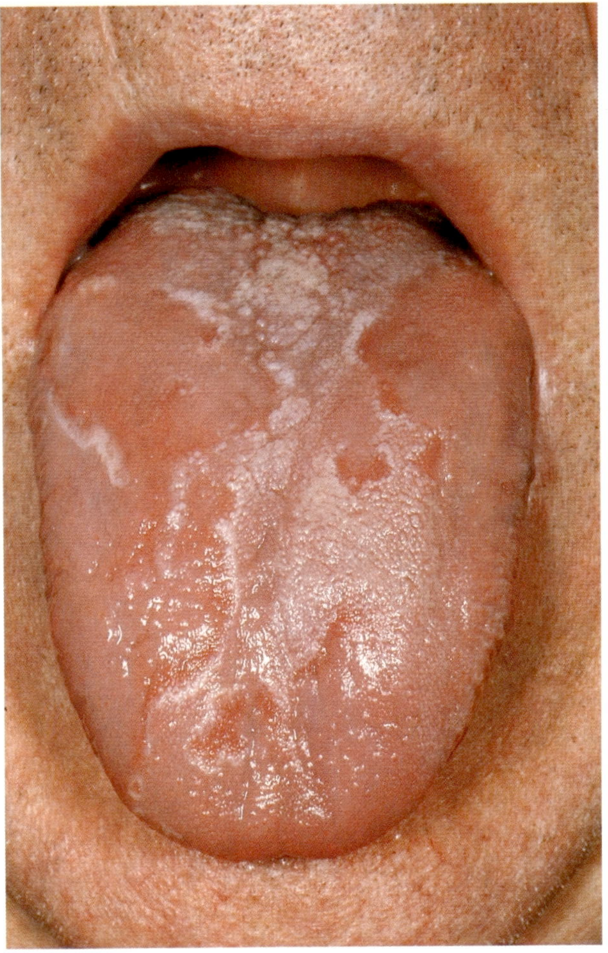

174

174 Circumscribed areas of whitish discoloration, partly in the shape of a garland, partly like a map, on the dorsum of the tongue. Lingual mucosa is otherwise slightly atrophic. (Male aged 54; clinically non-suspect)

175 Normal mucosa from the dorsum of the tongue, with papillae. Subepithelially, is collagenous fibrous tissue (stained green) with occasional blood vessels. *(Masson–Goldner)*

176 Mucosa from the tongue margin, with normal epithelium. Subepithelially, a slight increase in inflammatory cells can be seen.

177 Part of the basal epithelium showing a normal basal cell layer, with cellular polymorphism. Round cell infiltrates are slightly increased in the connective tissue.

Clinical management

Eliminate risk-factors. No treatment is required. Follow-up as part of general treatment.

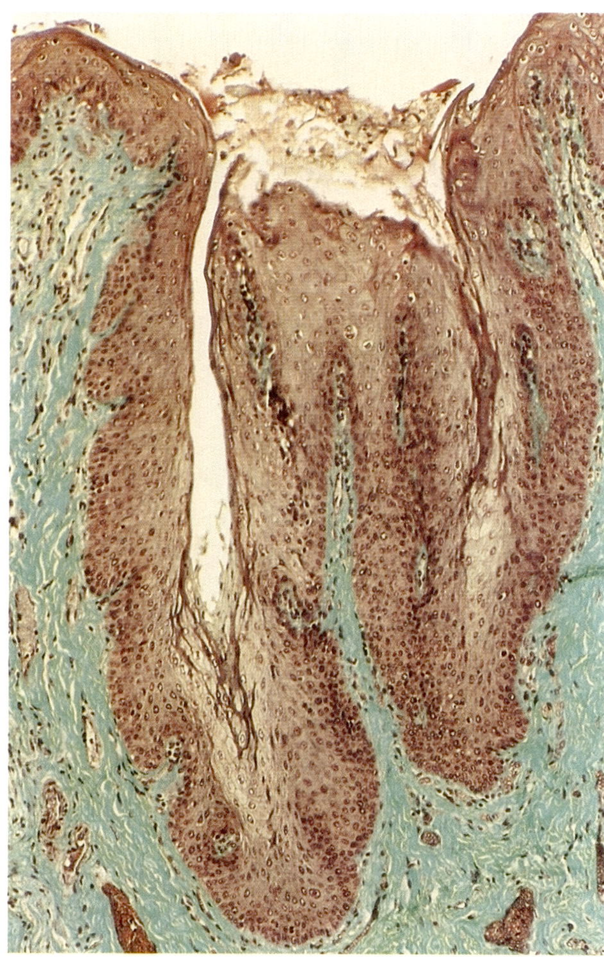

175

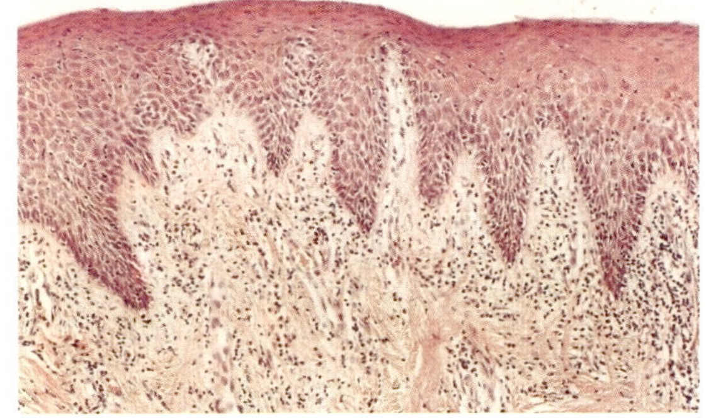

176

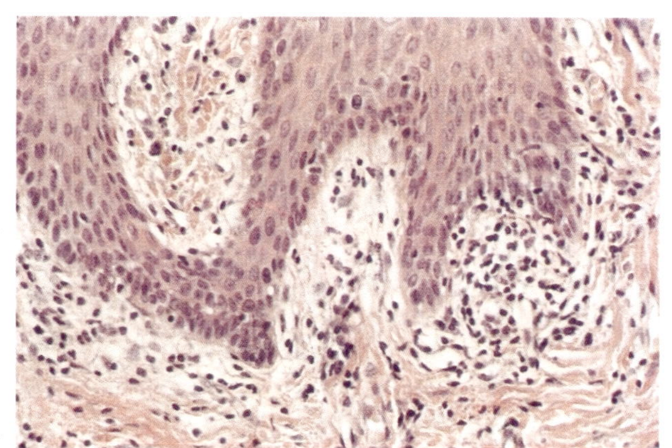

177

Median rhomboid glossitis (glossitis rhombica mediana)

This is a congenital anomaly in an area of separate embryological origin (tuberculum impar). The lesion is depressed or slightly raised, rhomboid and frequently associated with inflammatory changes which make it stand out more clearly. *Candida albicans* infection is common. Superficially, it is dark red in colour, but may also present with white patches. Histological examination shows epithelial hyperplasia but not dysplasia, with dendriform branching of the rete pegs a typical feature. Median rhomboid glossitis should be regarded as a harmless anomaly.

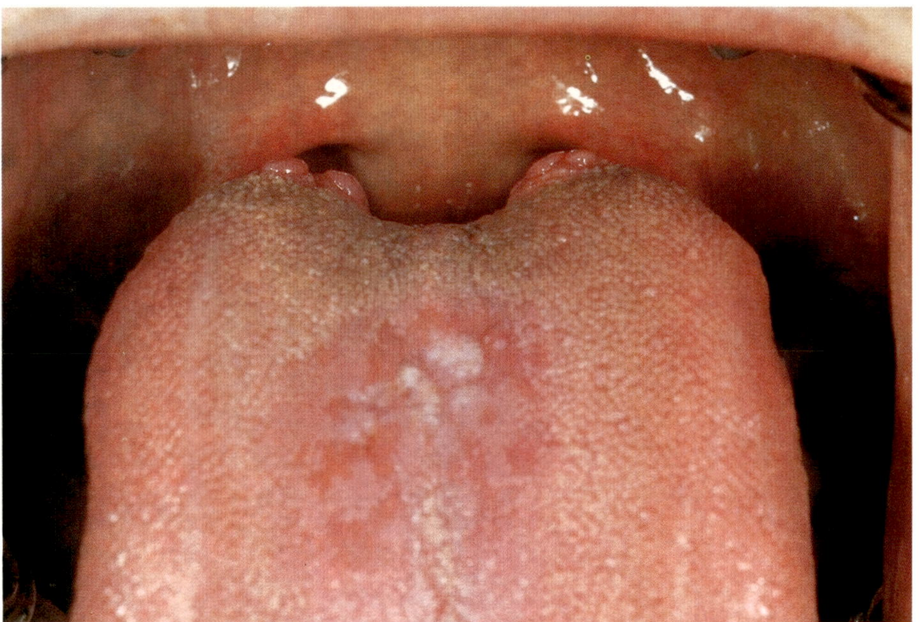

178

178 At the centre of the posterior third of the tongue, an oval reddish discoloration of the mucosa can be seen, its surface glabrous and atrophic. At the centre of the oval are homogeneous whitish patches that cannot be rubbed off. (Female aged 36; clinically non-suspect)

179 Epithelium shows irregularly formed rete pegs that are wide, deep and anastomosing. There is no dysplasia, but an inflammatory stroma infiltration can be seen, with inflammation extending into the epithelium.

180 Typical deep and branched rete pegs. No epithelial dysplasia. Inflammatory infiltration of the subepithelial tissue and epithelium.

181 Epithelial rete pegs show multiple pulvinate protrusions into connective tissue. There is marked basal cell hyperplasia in this area, but no dysplasia.

Clinical management

Undertake follow-up observation at intervals, as part of general treatment.

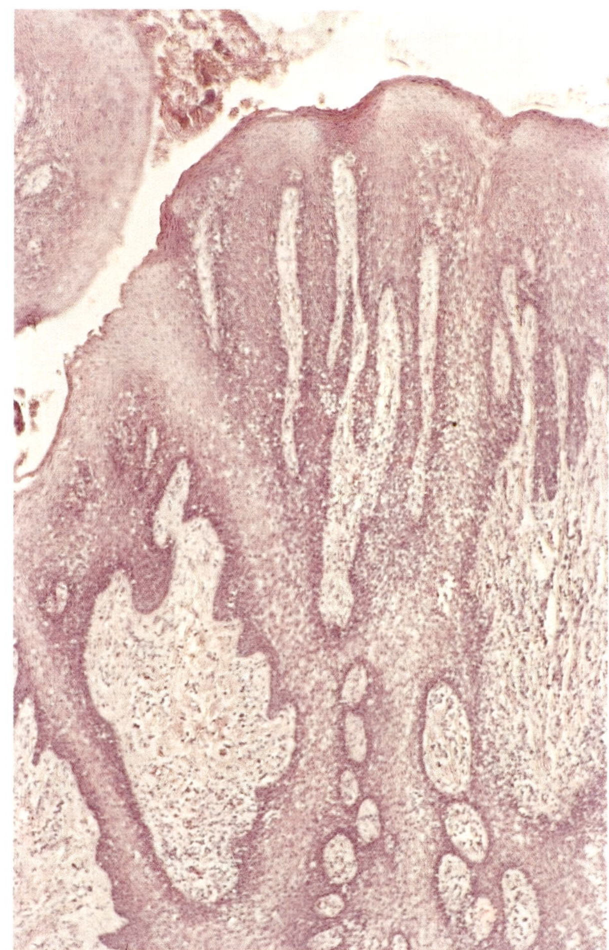

179

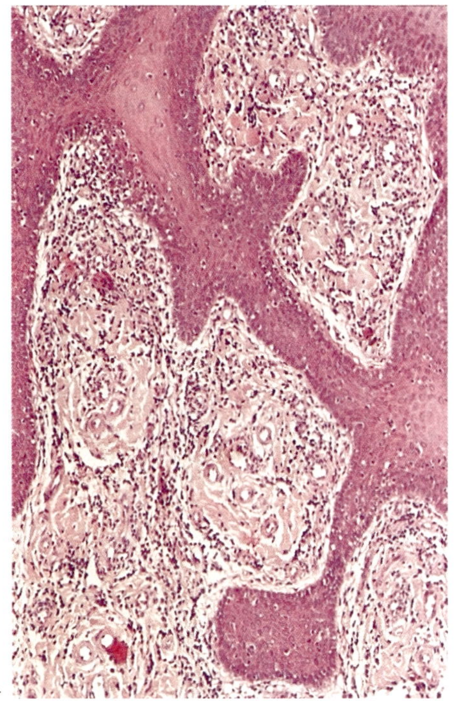

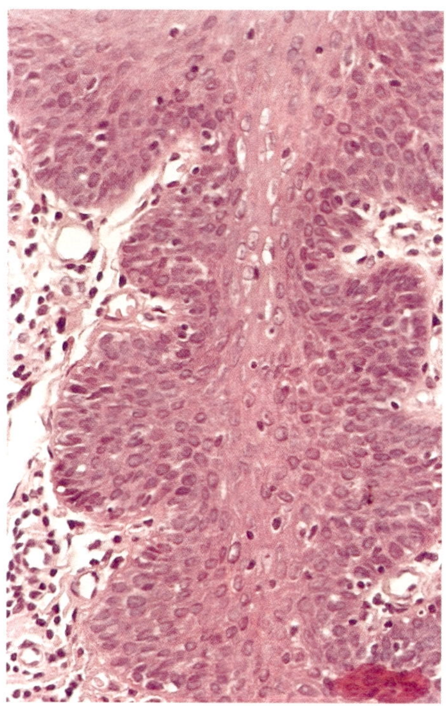

180
181►

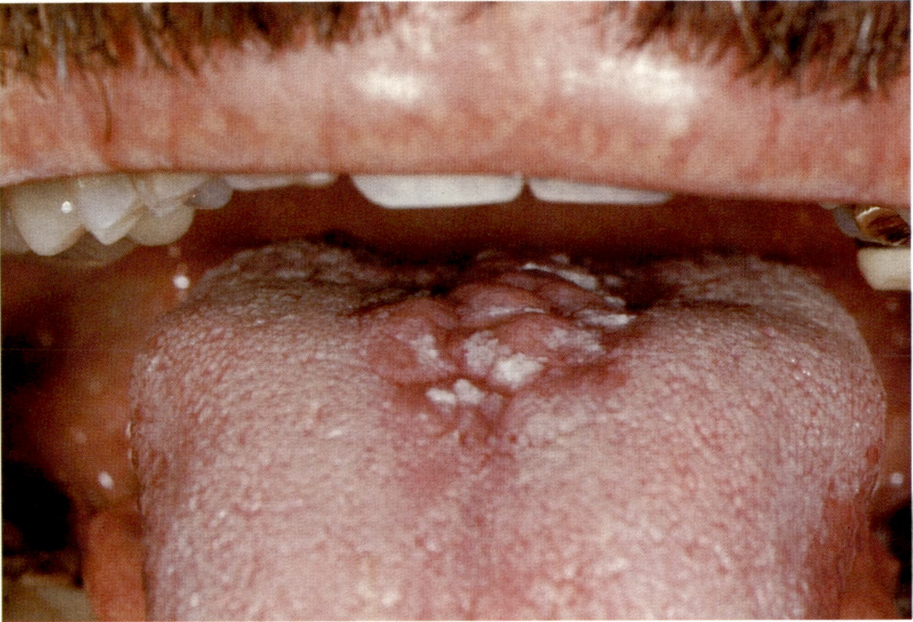

182

182 In the centre of the dorsum of the tongue, in the posterior third, a coarsely crenate reddened change in the mucosa can be seen, its surface fissured like a wall, with white patches that cannot be rubbed off. The area around this oval change shows a moderate degree of induration and is painful. (Male aged 36; clinically, carcinoma based on median rhomboid glossitis a definite possibility)

183 Superficial parts of the epithelium are irregular, with exophytic papillomatous projections. Rete pegs are extended and anastomosing. There is definite focal acanthosis, and the stroma is fibrotic. *(Masson–Goldner)*

184 Long, drawn rete pegs and inflammatory sponginess of epithelium. Superficially, there is irregular desquamation and inflammatory infiltration but no indication of *Candida albicans* infection. Subepithelial connective tissue contains round cell infiltrates.

185 High-power micrograph of basal epithelium. A dense inflammatory infiltration is clearly discernible in the region of the basal layer and lower prickle cell layer.

Clinical management

Admission to hospital for excision into healthy tissue and histological examination. In this case (Figures **182** to **185**) examination confirmed a median rhomboid glossitis with a high degree of inflammation, but no carcinoma or dysplasia. Follow-up as part of general treatment measures.

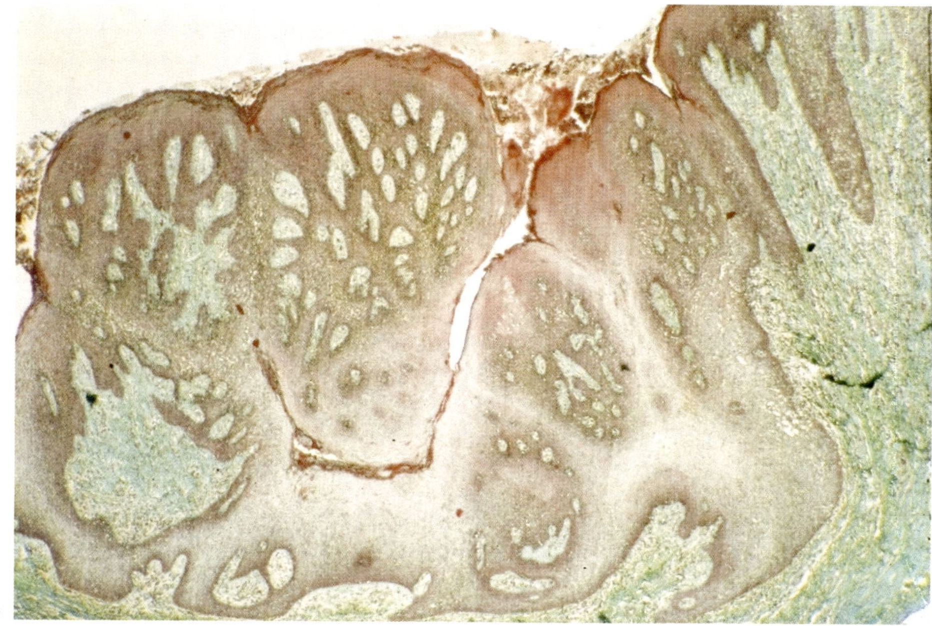

183

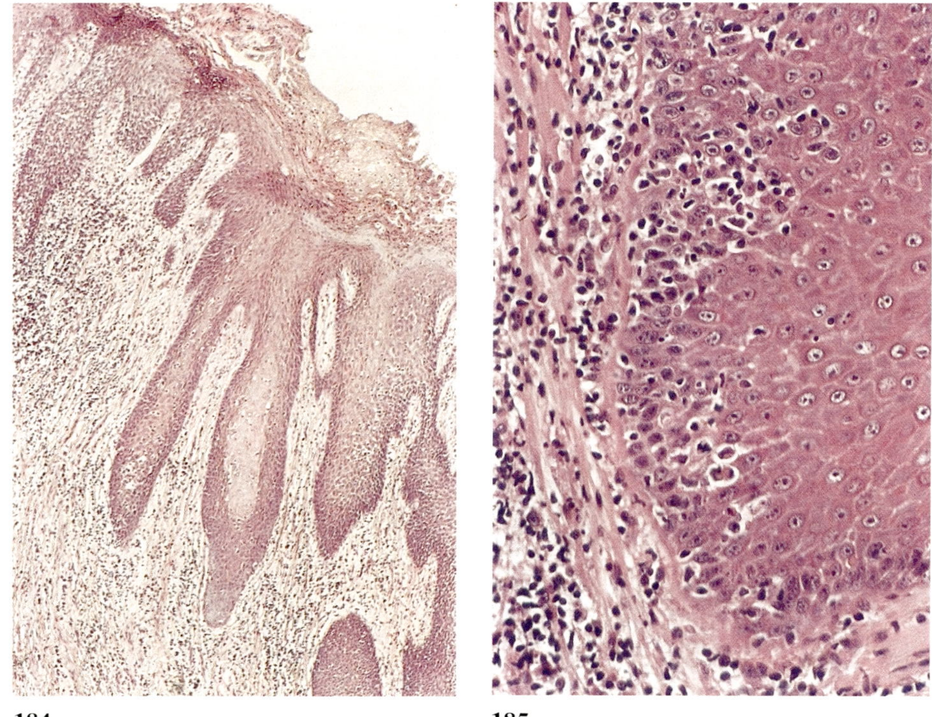

184

185

White changes in the mucosa arising from inflammatory lesions

A number of inflammatory lesions affecting the oral mucosa may also involve reactive epithelial hyperplasia, usually in the marginal areas. On inspection, they present as whitish changes in the mucosa. Experienced practitioners will, as a rule, diagnose the underlying condition and institute treatment. The mucosal changes will then disappear with the inflammation.

Symptomatic leukoplakias of this type may also be seen with cheilitis, a condition of uncertain origin, and granulamatous glossitis (Melkersson–Rosenthal syndrome).

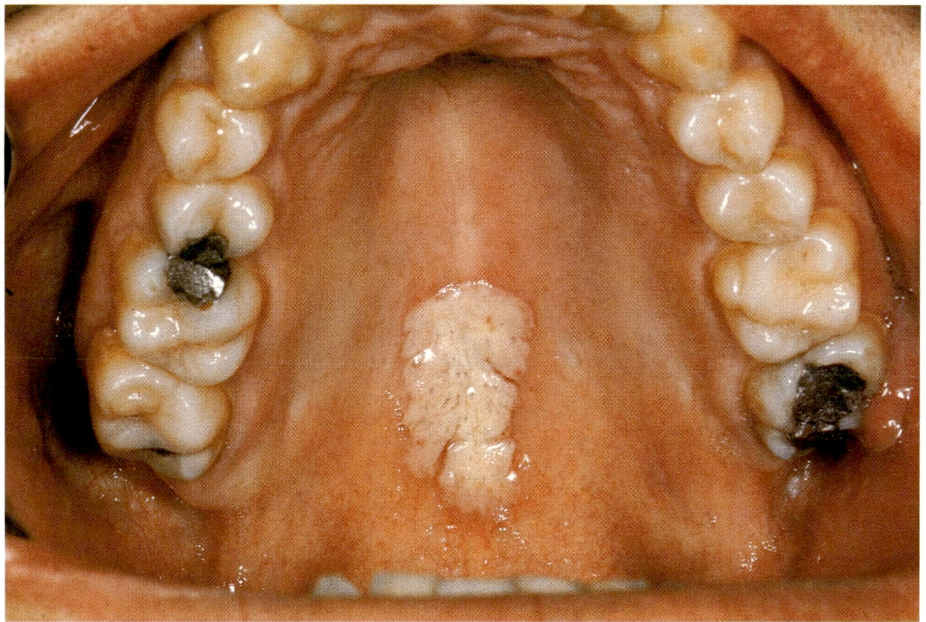

186

186 Whitish verrucous change in the mucosa, with narrow reddish margins, that cannot be rubbed off, in the central part of the hard palate, with transition to the soft palate. (Male aged 32; clinically non-suspect)

187 Highly inflammatory spongy epithelium showing superficial erosions and fibrin deposits interspersed with granulocytes. The stroma also shows dense inflammatory infiltration.

188 Spongy epithelium with dense granulocytic infiltration.

189 Ulcerative epithelial defect with superficial fibrin deposits and dense round cell infiltration of connective tissue enclosing granulocytes.

Clinical management

Diagnosis is based on the history, general dermatological examination and serological studies. Biopsy should be taken only in cases of doubt.

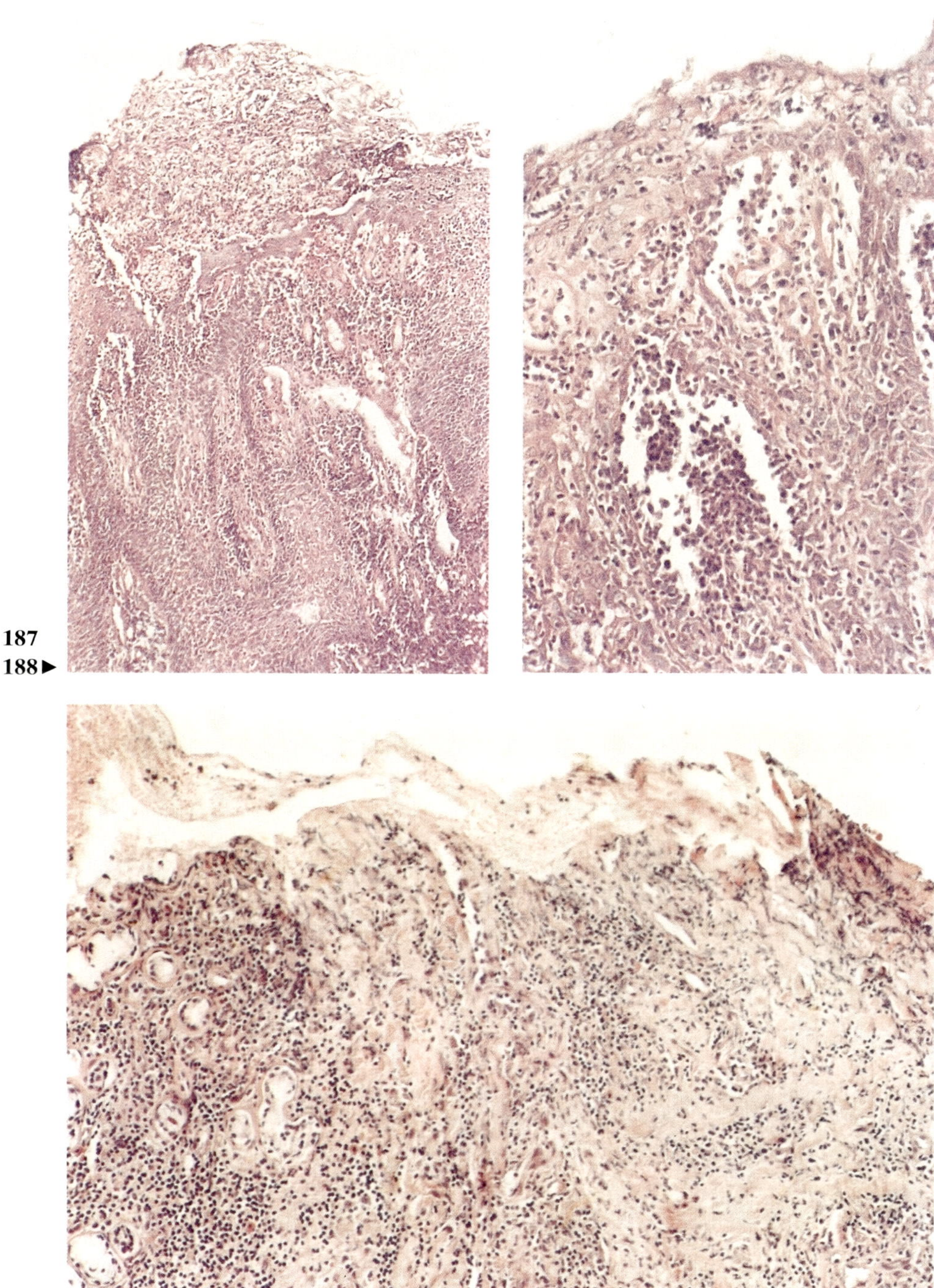

187
188►

189

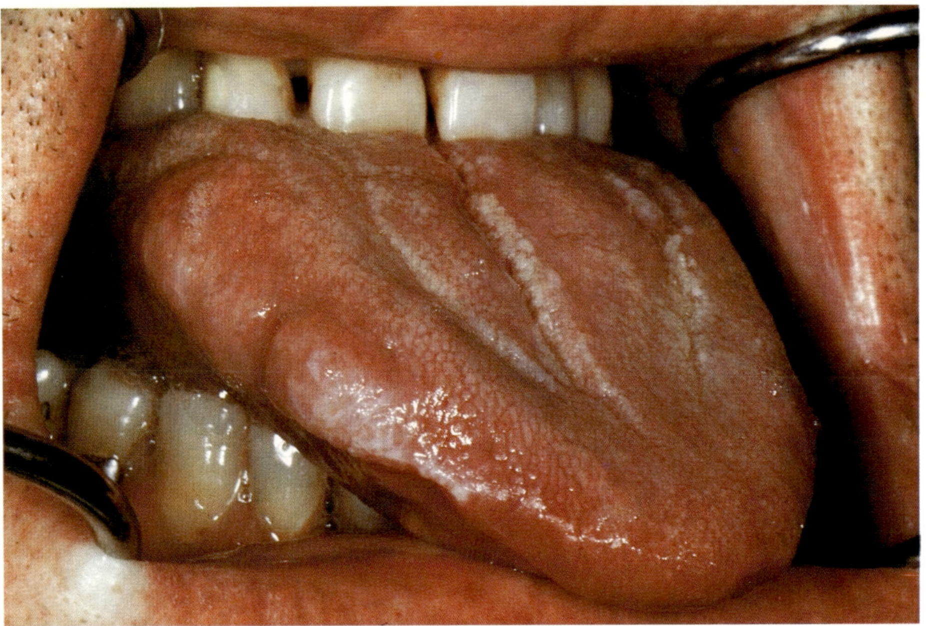

190

190 White to pale grey striated changes overlying solid nodular indurations in the margin and dorsum of the tongue. (Male aged 57; clinically, local condition suspected)

191 Superficially normal epithelium with low-degree acanthosis and parakeratosis. Subepithelially, fibrotic connective tissue can be seen, with collagen fibres in whorls and bundles among which small granulamatous inflammatory infiltrates are embedded.

192 Collagen fibrous tissue, thinly scattered with small granulomata.

193 High-power micrograph of two small inflammatory cell granulomata. Nodular accretions of inflammatory cells can be seen, consisting predominantly of lymphocytes, but also of histiocytes and occasional narrow epithelioid cells.

Clinical management

Diagnosis can be made as part of general examination (dermatological examination), and histology verified by biopsy.

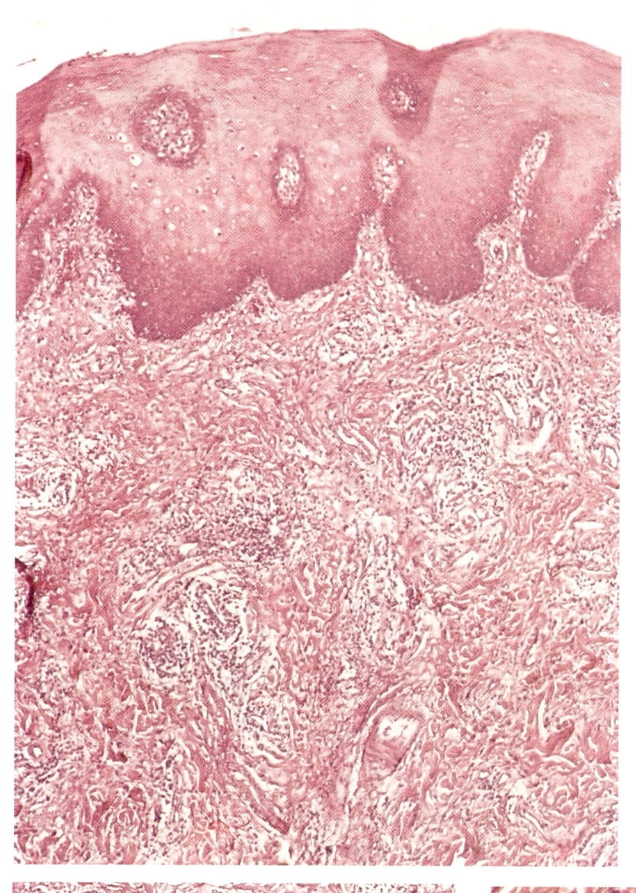

191

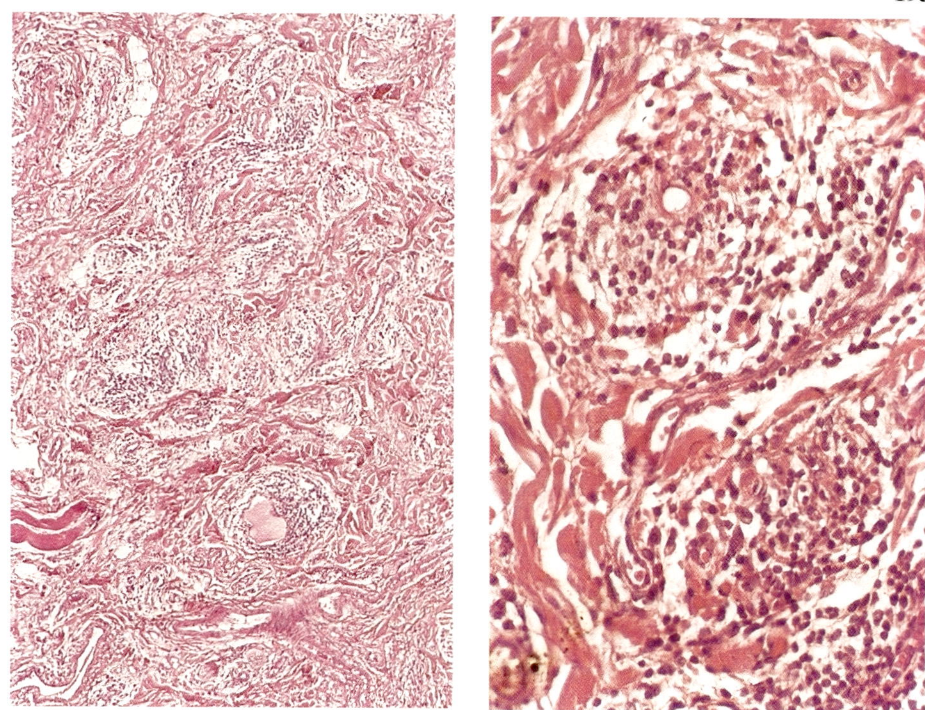

192

193

Non-malignant ulceration of the mucosa

Non-neoplastic ulceration in the mucosa is usually inflammatory or traumatic in origin. Typically, such ulcers usually heal rapidly. If an ulcer persists and shows no tendency to heal when conservative treatment has been given for a maximum of 10 days, malignancy must be suspected, even when there is no marginal infiltration. Admission to hospital and histological examination of a fast-frozen section are absolutely essential in such cases.

Relatively large single aphthous ulcers may also appear suspicious, particularly as the surrounding tissues may be indurated. They are very painful, however, with a characteristically short history and tend to heal rapidly, so that in the majority of cases the correct diagnosis presents no problem.

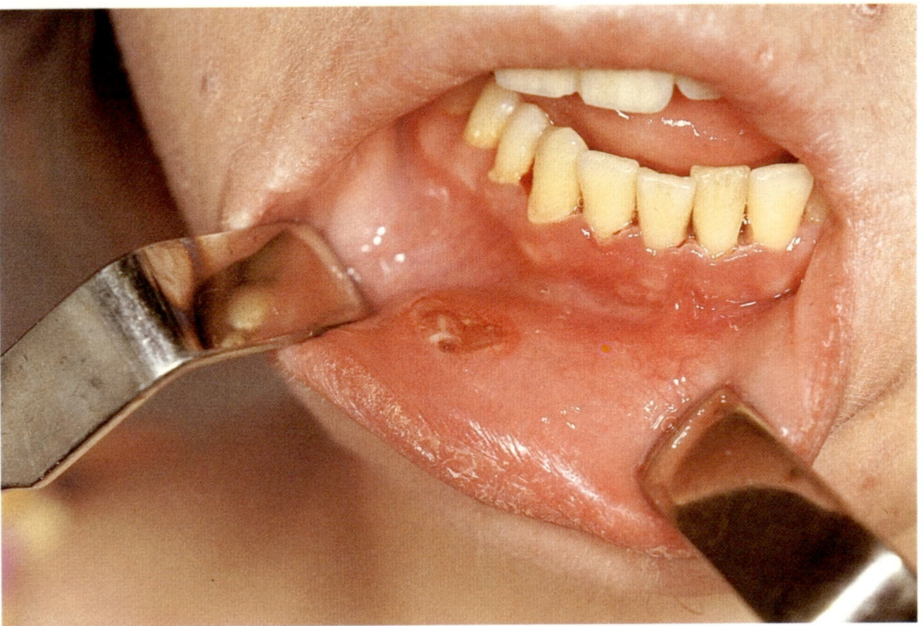

194

194 A punchhole-like ulcer, 1 × 1cm in area, with hard, painfree margins and indolent swelling of regional submandibular lymph node. (Female aged 22; clinically, a malignant local lesion is highly suspected)

195 Superficially, epithelium is very spongy due to inflammation. There are fibrin deposits and dense round cell infiltrates in the connective tissue.

196 Ulcerated lesion with capillary buds, round cell infiltrates and granulocytic infiltrates.

197 Seromucous glands deep down, with dense lymphocytic inflammatory infiltration in the surrounding area.

Clinical management

In view of the relative youth of the patient, relevant history should be taken. Primary syphilis is a possible cause. Appropriate dermatological examination and serological studies should be made. Primary syphilis was established. If this had not been the case, histological examination to exclude carcinoma would have been essential.

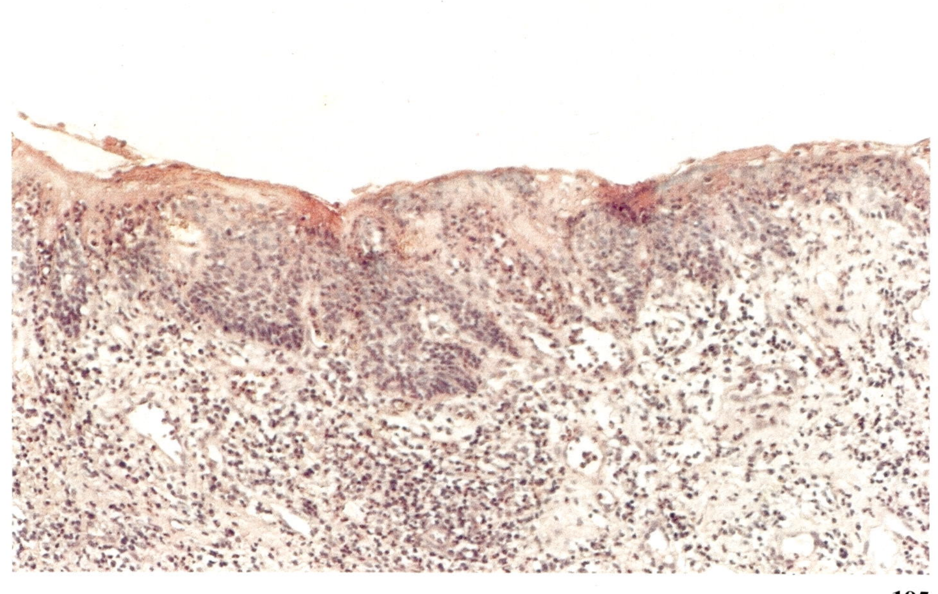

195

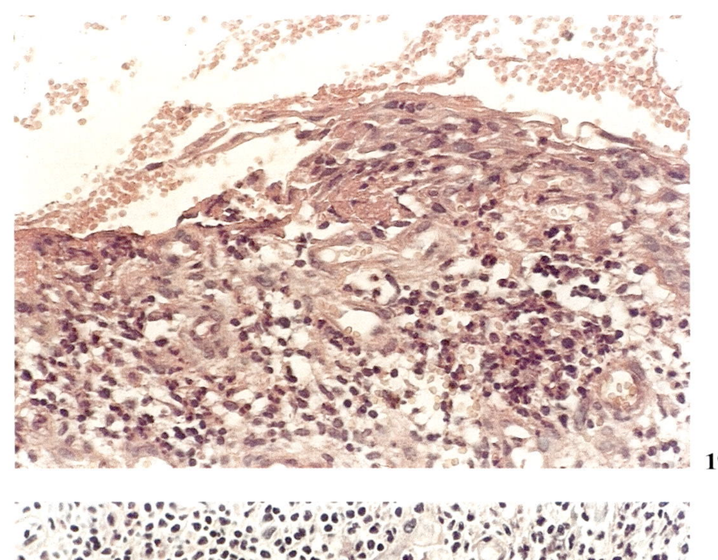

196

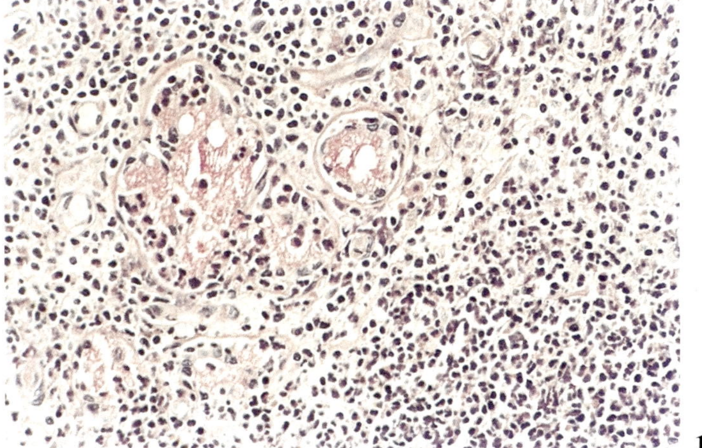

197

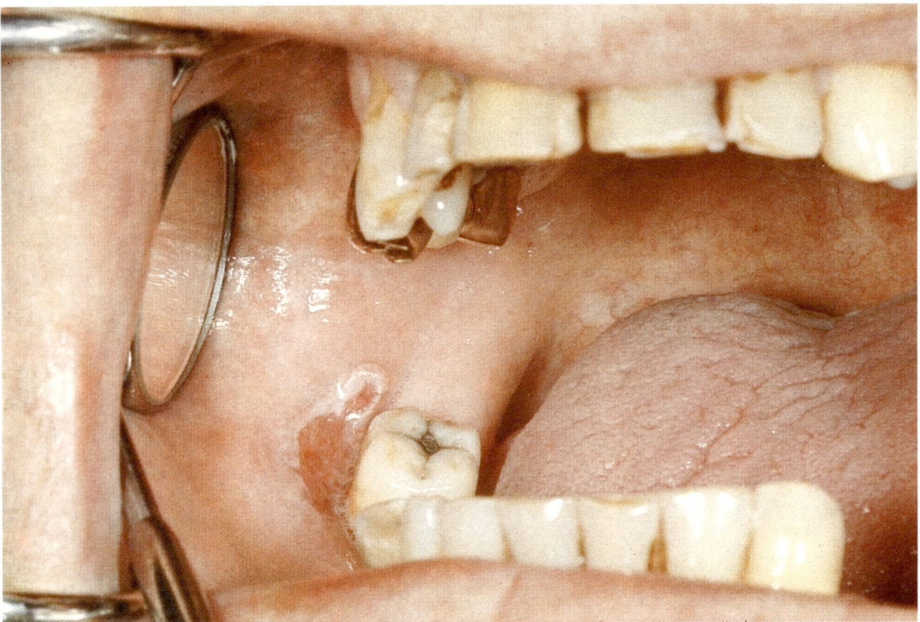

198

198 A circumscribed erosion, not infiltrating, with whitish changes where it borders onto healthy mucosa, immediately adjacent to tooth 48. (Male aged 47, in good health; clinically, primarily non-suspect, because of relation to inflamed periodontium)

199 Broad ulcerative epithelial defect with superficial fibrin deposits interspersed with granulocytes. Incipient cicatrisation can be seen deep down. Residual epithelium is discernible in the right marginal area.

200 Dense inflammatory infiltration deep down, with enclosure of numerous lymphocytes and plasma cells.

201 Regenerated epithelium showing enlarged and hyperchromic nuclei.

Clinical management

Eliminate risk-factors, undertake conservative treatment and short-term follow-up observation for a maximum of 10 days. If there is no regression after that period, excision biopsy is essential, with further treatment dependent on histological findings. In this case (Figures **198** to **201**), the lesion healed with conservative treatment.

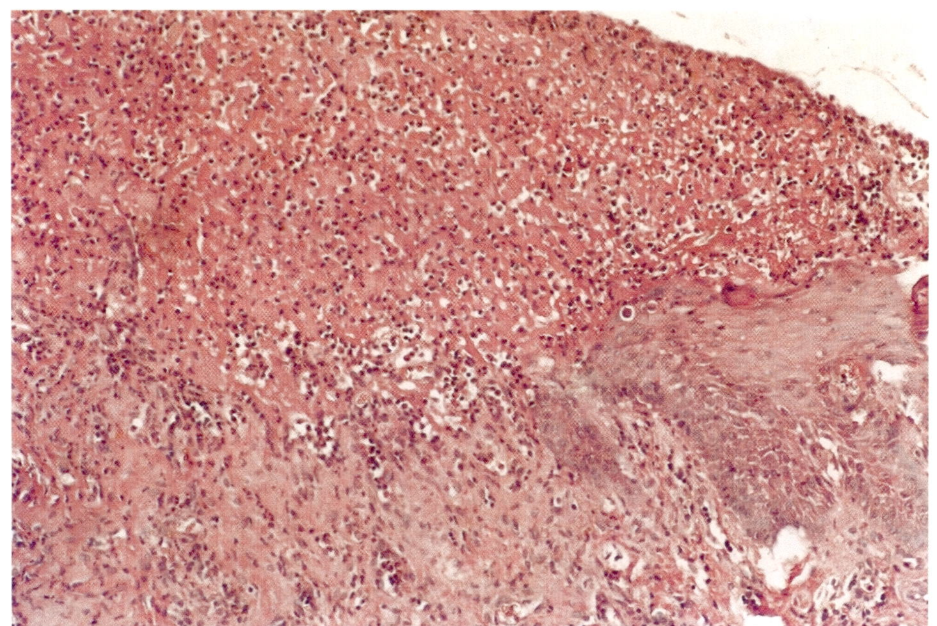

199

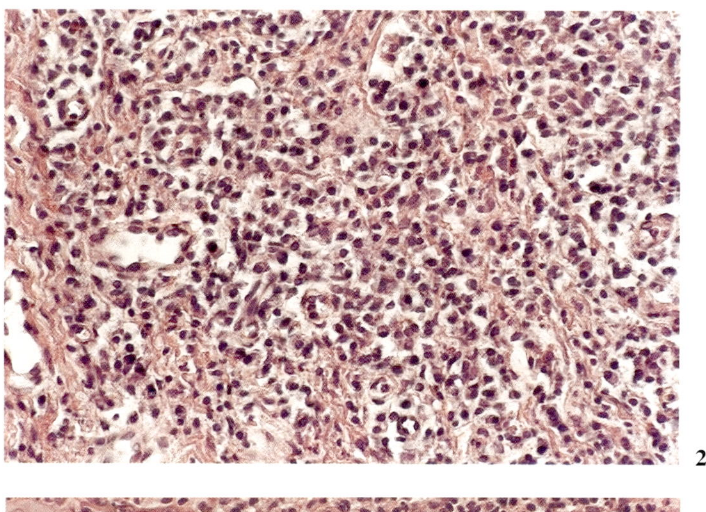

200

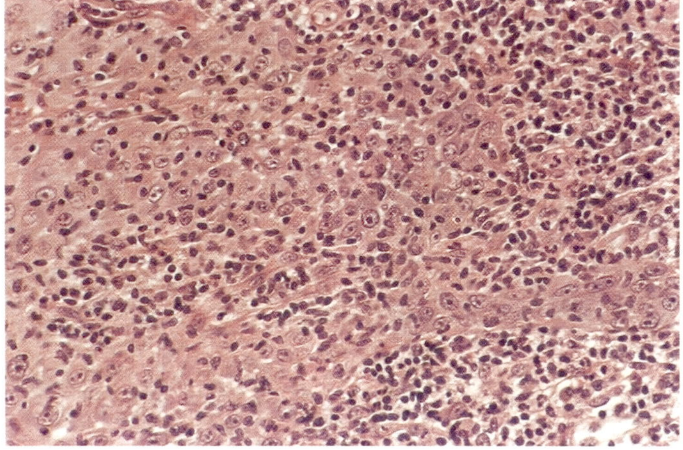

201

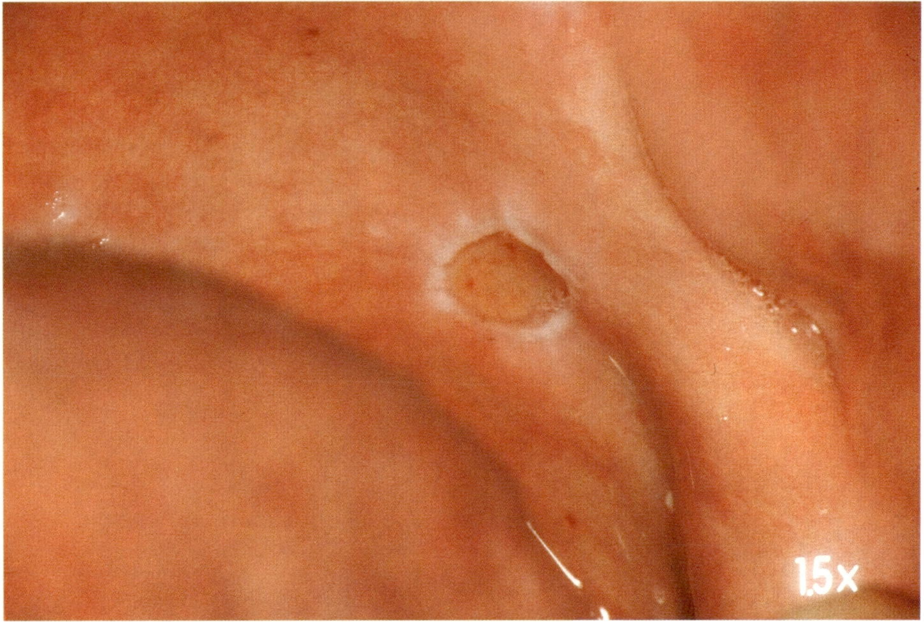

202

202 Sharply circumscribed painful erosion, 5 × 5mm in area, in the mucosa of the velum, adjacent to the pterygomandibular fold. There is no marginal infiltration, but a slight degree of whitish discoloration can be seen in the margins. (Male aged 54; clinically non-suspect)

203 A punchhole-like ulcerated lesion, with dense inflammatory infiltration in the region of the ulcer. The marginal area shows regenerating epithelium.

204 Part of the marginal area of the ulcer, with regenerating epithelium. Slight nuclear hyperchromatism and increased mitotic figures can be seen. The epithelium is clearly inflamed and spongy.

205 High-power micrograph of epithelial cone showing low-degree nuclear hyperchromatism and increased number of mitotic figures. These areas show slight reactive epithelial dysplasia and increased mitosis, indicative of epithelial regeneration and not precancerous dysplasia.

Clinical management

Conservative treatment is indicated, combined with treatment of general infectious condition, if present. Histological examination is only necessary if the condition persists or increases.

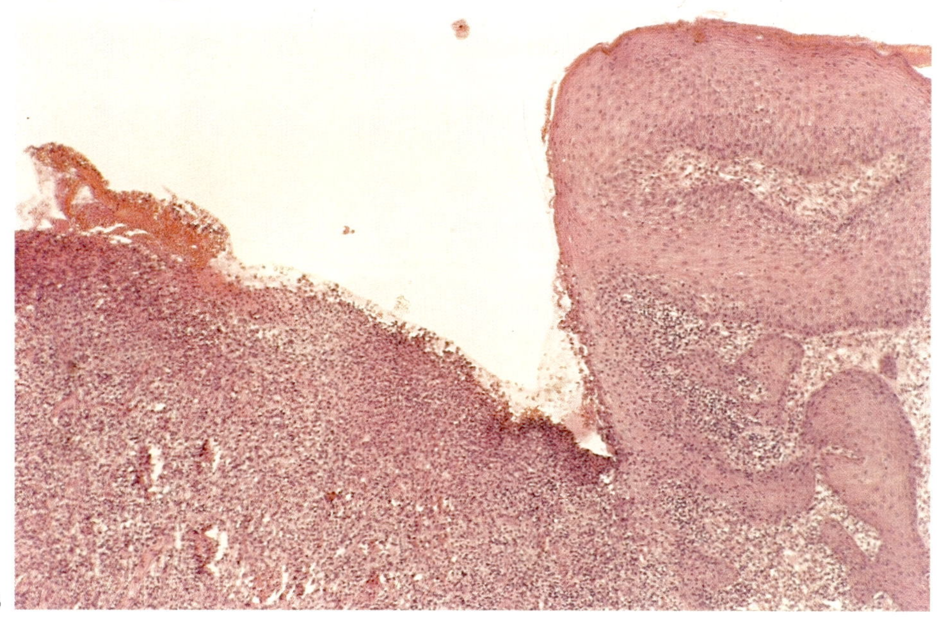

203

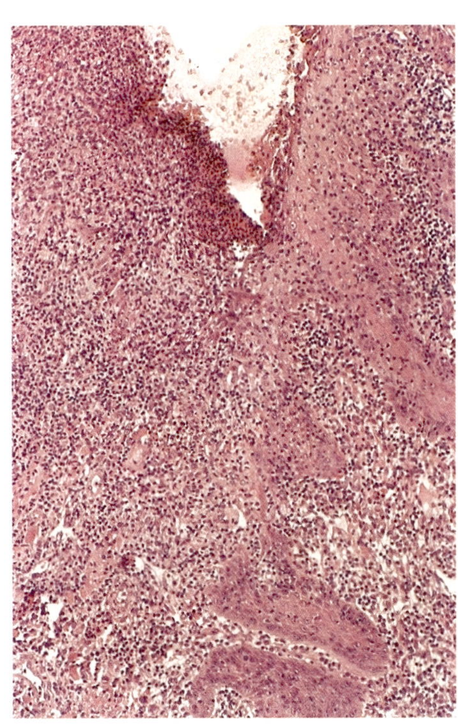

204

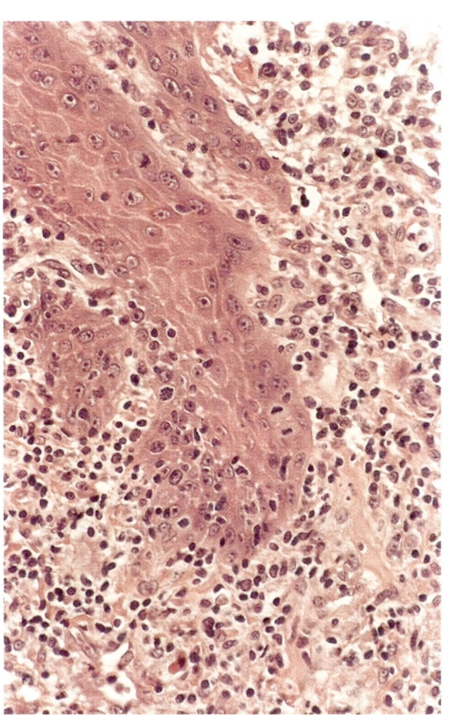

205

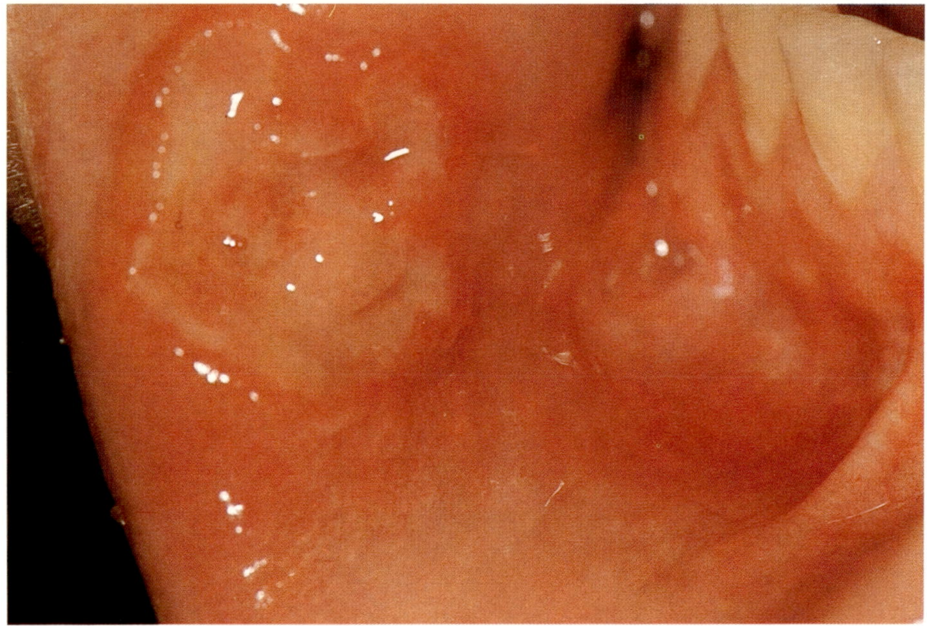

206

206 A sharply circumscribed painful erosion in the lower lip, with slightly infiltrated margins. Superficially, whitish fibrinous deposits can be seen. (Male aged 15; clinically some doubt because of marginal infiltration)

207 Surface of ulcer showing necrosis and dense, mainly granulocytic inflammatory infiltrates.

208 Deeper down in the ulcer, granulating inflammation with ectatic capillaries, capillary buds and fibroblastic proliferation has occurred.

209 Highly inflamed, spongy epithelium in marginal area of the ulcer. Nuclei are enlarged and slightly hyperchromatic.

Clinical management

Excision biopsy and histological examination should be done. In this case (Figures **206** to **209**) a nonspecific ulcer was found, with nothing to indicate malignancy. Subsequently more aphthae developed. Conservative treatment is indicated, combined with treatment of general infectious disease, if present.

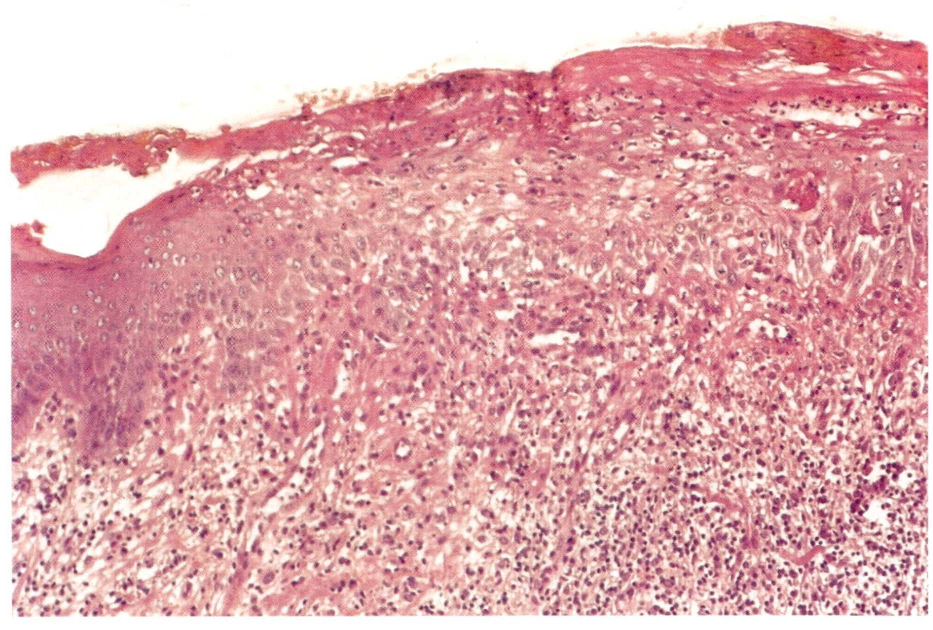

215

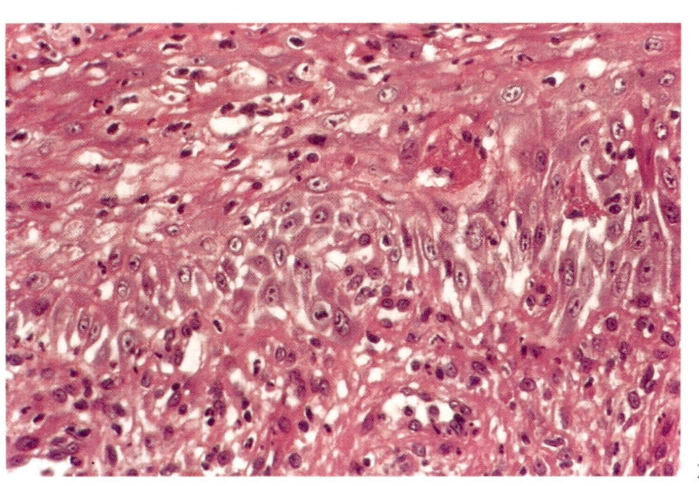

216

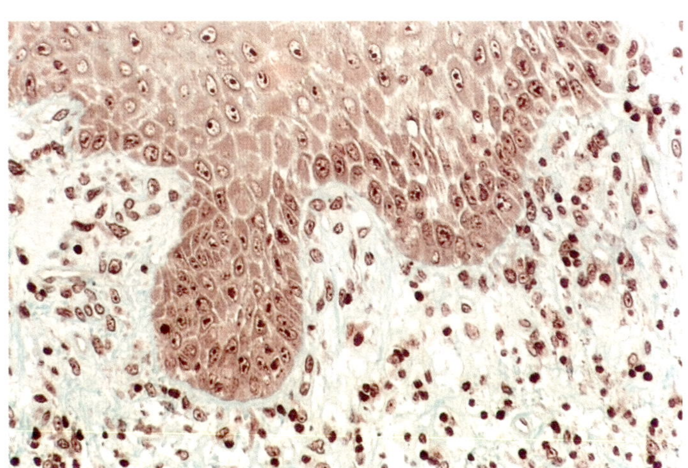

217

Fordyce spots (heterotopic sebaceous glands)

The occurrence of sebaceous glands in the region of the buccal mucosa is a heterotopia of developmental origin and is a harmless anomaly. It presents as yellow or whitish spots of very characteristic appearance that only the inexperienced will mistake for leukoplakic lesions.

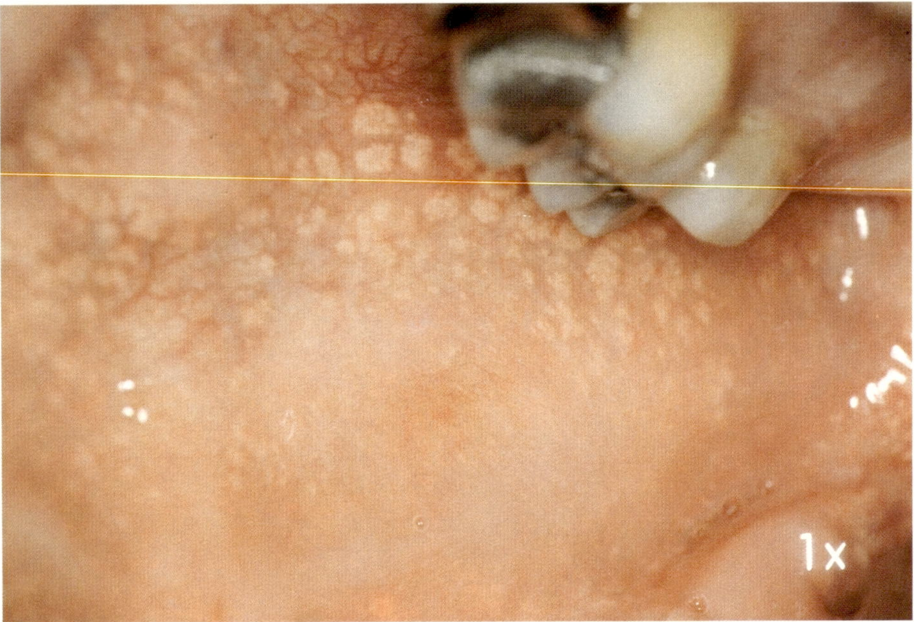

218

218 Multiple raised yellowish changes in an otherwise normal mucosal surface, with no ulceration or infiltration. (Male patient aged 38, in good health; clinically unequivocal and non-suspect)

219 Superficially, epithelium is normal with a low degree of basal cell hyperplasia. In the underlying connective tissue, a typical lobulated sebaceous gland can be seen.

220 High-power micrograph of the sacculated sebaceous gland showing typical bright, loose-structured cell body.

Clinical management

No treatment is required.

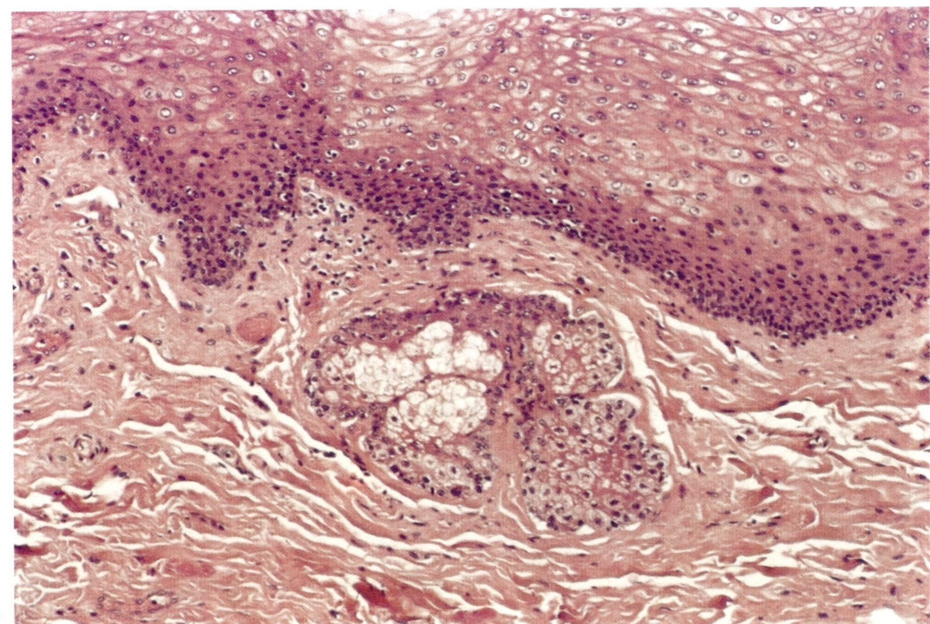

219

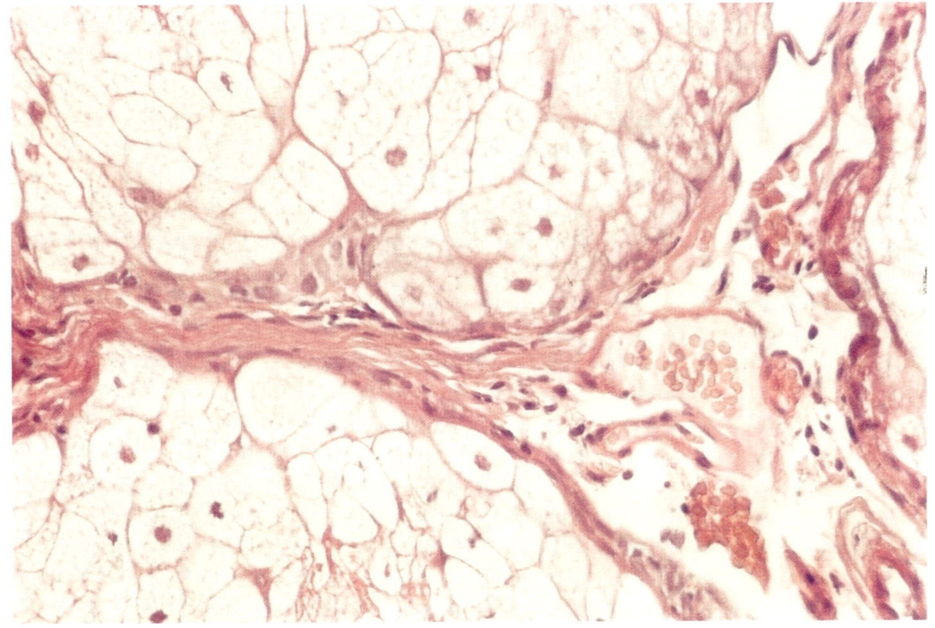

220

Lichen planus

Lichen planus is a dermoepidermal condition of unknown origin involving degeneration of the basal layer. On the external skin it presents as polygonal, slightly raised papules that are livid red in colour. In the oral mucosa, especially of the cheeks, whitish striated or reticular configurations appear (reticular type), which may also be confluent. Dark-red areas with epithelial atrophy, erosions and bullous lesions have also been noted. These appearances differentiate the condition from leukoplakia and erythroplakia.

Characteristic histological features are saw-toothed, shallow rete pegs, degeneration (liquefaction) of basal cells, subepithelial oedema with vacuoles forming between stroma and epithelium, and a band-like inflammatory infiltration subepithelially consisting almost entirely of lymphocytes.

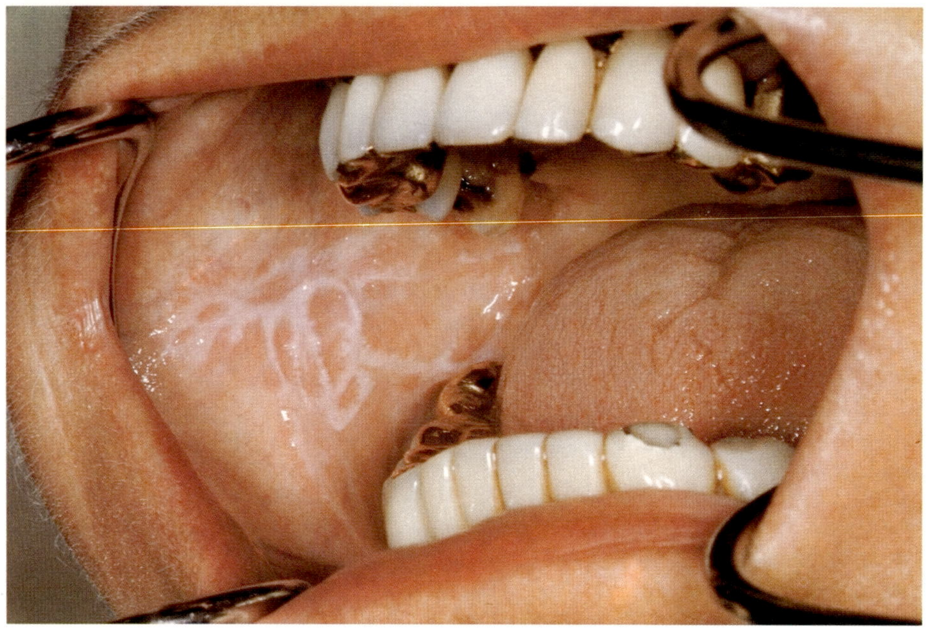

221

221 Fine whitish, filigree-like striations on the posterior buccal mucosa, that cannot be rubbed off. There is no infiltration or ulceration. (Female aged 61; clinically non-suspect)

222 Epithelium showing typical narrow, partly saw-toothed rete pegs. The prickle cell layer is normal in appearance, the basal cell layer is poorly delimited, and there is a dense, predominantly lymphocytic infiltrate in stroma.

223 Epithelial rete peg with no recognisable basal cell layer, inflamed and spongy surrounding areas, with dense lymphocytic infiltrates.

224 Basal epithelium showing degeneration of basal cells and vacuoles in this area. Lymphocytic infiltrates can be seen subepithelially.

Clinical management

Conservative treatment is indicated. Further observation should be made as part of general treatment. In case of doubt, biopsy will confirm the diagnosis.

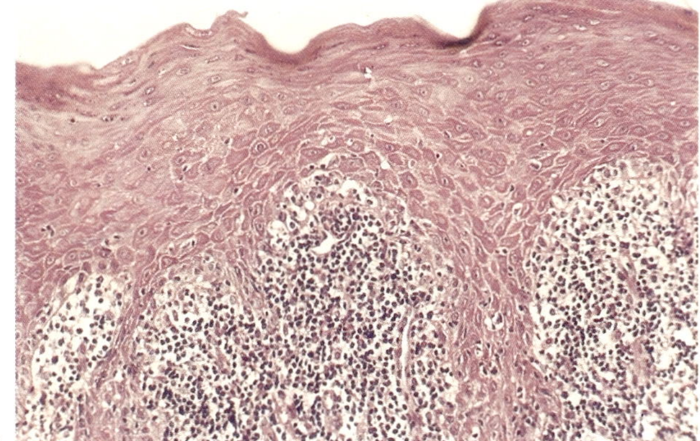

222

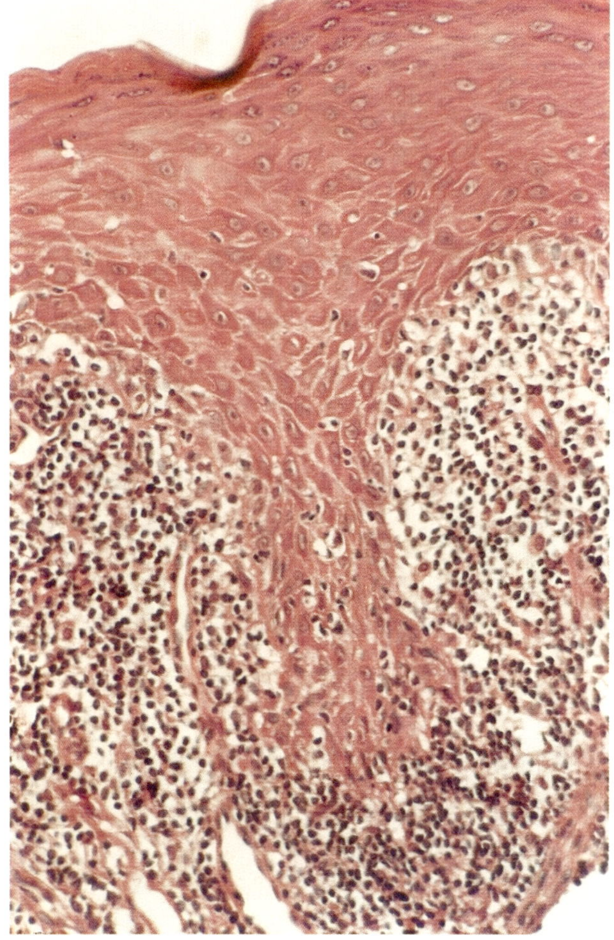

223

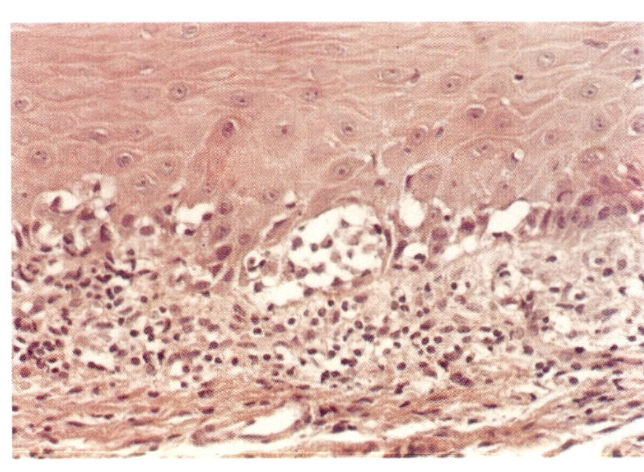

224

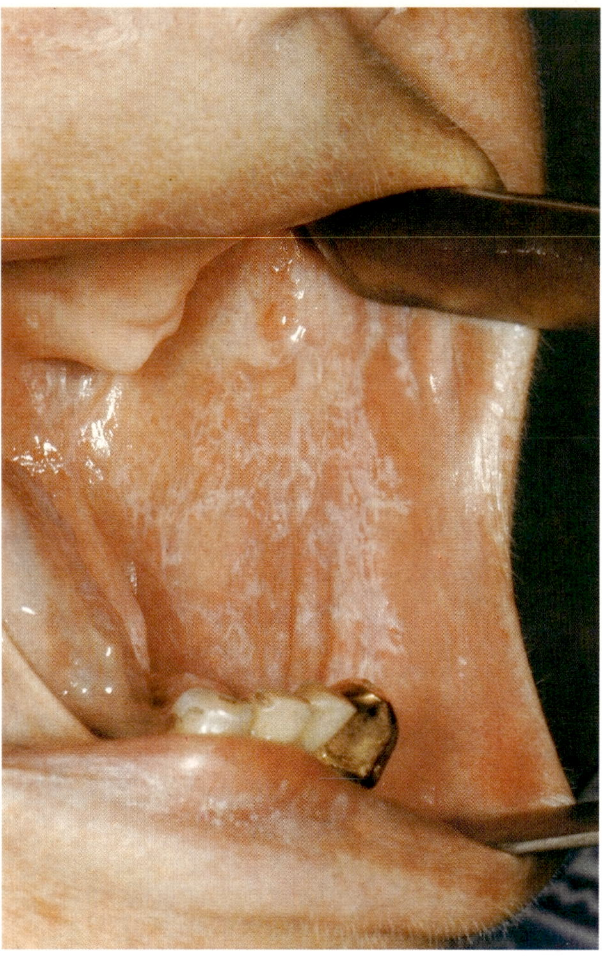

225

225 Extensive, delicately branching, filigree-like, whitish discoloration of buccal mucosa, with no redness, infiltration or ulceration. (Female aged 61; clinically non-suspect)

226 Superficial epithelium showing normal stratification and orthokeratosis. Basally, rete pegs are pointed, the basal cell layer is not discernible, and narrow spaces are present between epithelium and stroma.

227 Basal epithelium with basal cell layer absent and rete pegs showing saw-toothed extension. There are narrow spaces between epithelium and stroma and lymphocytic infiltrations subepithelially.

228 Epithelium is largely detached in this area; there are ectatic capillaries in the connective tissue and lymphocytic infiltrates in the surrounding area.

Clinical management

Conservative treatment is indicated with follow-up observation as part of general treatment. In cases of doubt, biopsy will confirm the diagnosis.

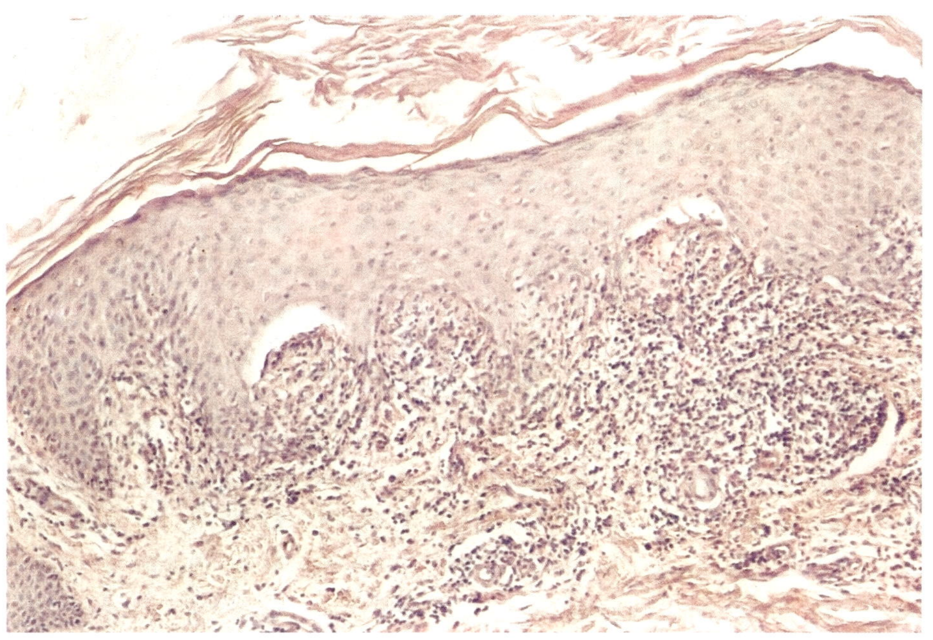

226

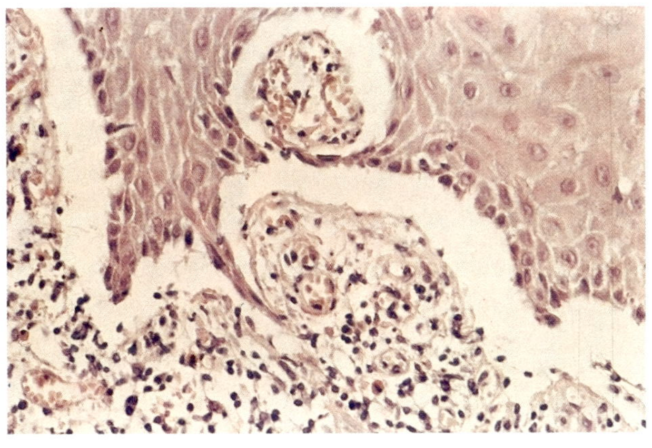

227

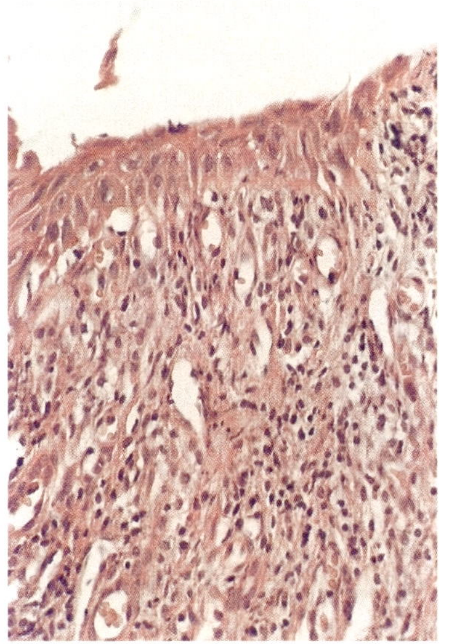

228

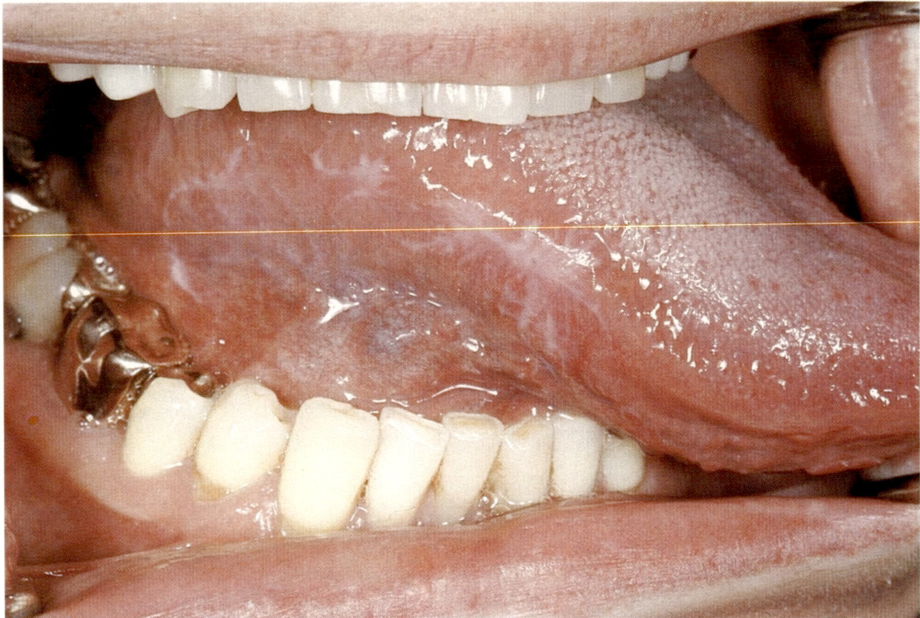

229

229 Typical fine, striated, fern-like, whitish markings in the margin of the tongue. There is no infiltration and oral hygiene is good. (Male aged 44; clinically non-suspect)

230 Epithelium showing focal acanthosis and a low degree of hyperparakeratosis. Basally, rete pegs are extended to a point. Dense lymphocytic infiltrates are present in the stroma.

231 Basal epithelium with indistinct basal cell layer and normal prickle cell layer. Increased numbers of interepithelial lymphocytes can be seen and there is dense inflammatory infiltration of the subepithelial stroma.

Clinical management

Conservative treatment is indicated with follow-up as part of general treatment. If the lesion increases, biopsy should be undertaken to confirm the diagnosis.

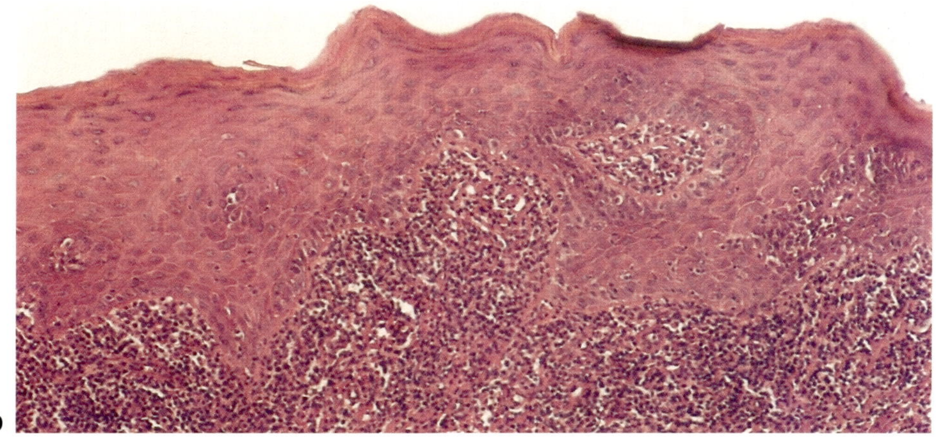

230

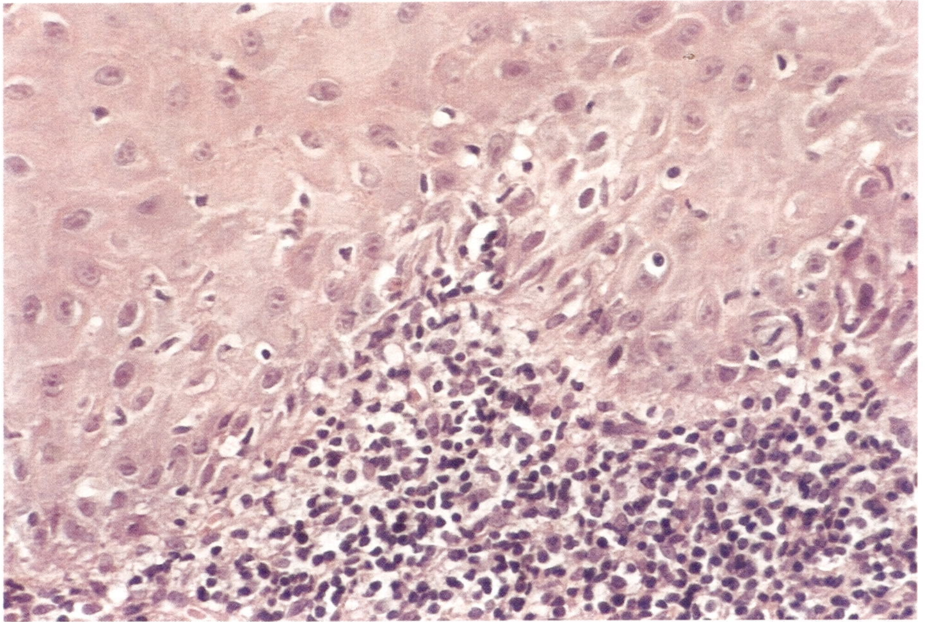

231

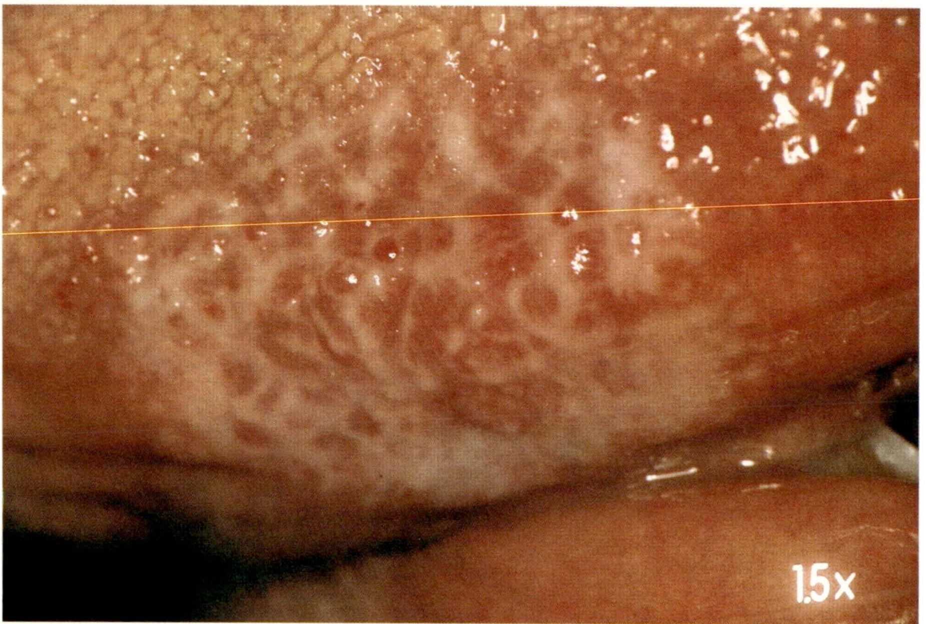

232

232 Reticulated whitish changes in the oral mucosa, with no ulceration or infiltration. (Female aged 75; clinically, lichen planus suspected)

233 Epithelium showing increased basal cone formation, low-degree acanthosis and hyperparakeratosis. An inflammatory reaction has occurred in the stroma.

234 Epithelial cones with clearly enlarged hyperchromic nuclei.

235 Polar arrangement of basal cells is absent, and prickle cells show irregular maturation and dyskeratosis.

Clinical management

The margin of the tongue being a high-risk area, biopsy should be taken for histological examination. In this case (Figures **232** to **235**) lichen planus was not confirmed but a high degree of epithelial dysplasia was found. Total excision into healthy tissue was, therefore, absolutely essential. Follow-up observation as for carcinoma is required, in the oncological clinic of the hospital.

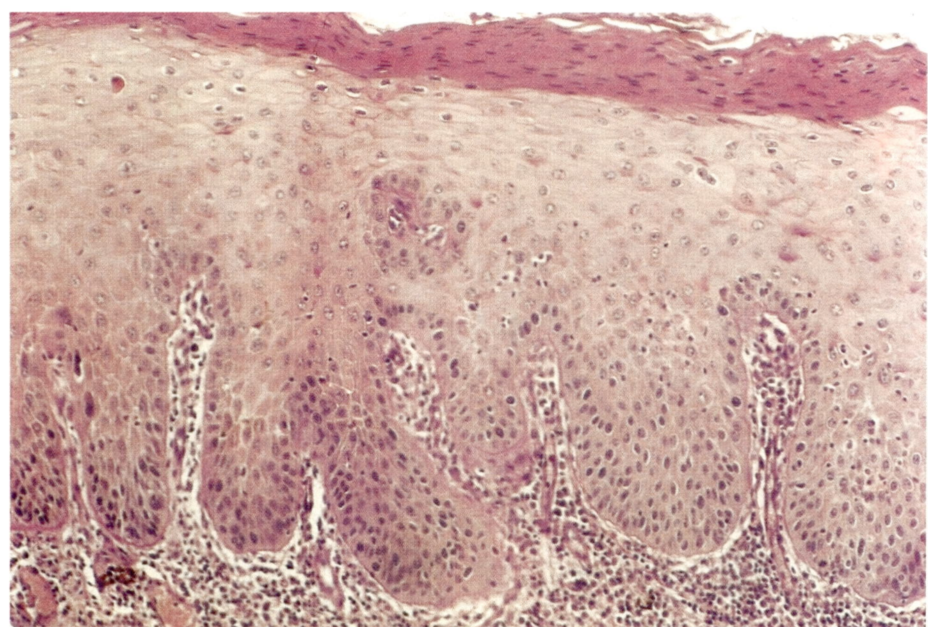

233

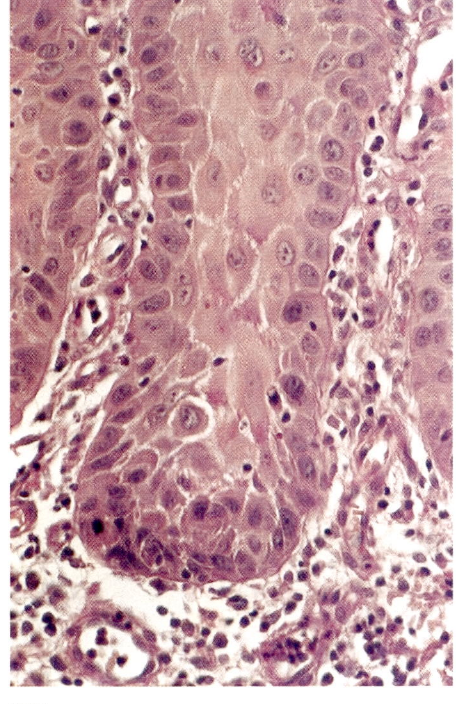

234

235

Pemphigus vulgaris

Pemphigus is a bullous dermatosis characterised by acantholysis (dissolution of the intercellular bridges in the prickle cell layer) provoked by antibodies to structural elements in the epithelium. Intraepithelial vesicles are produced. Similar changes may also affect the oral mucosa. The bullae tend to rupture after a short time and are then seen as red, bleeding erosions, frequently with whitish changes in the surrounding mucosa.

The histological features are characteristic – acantholysis, intraepithelial suprabasal vesicles and, in the marginal surrounding erosions, rows of still extant basal cells, while the upper layers are missing.

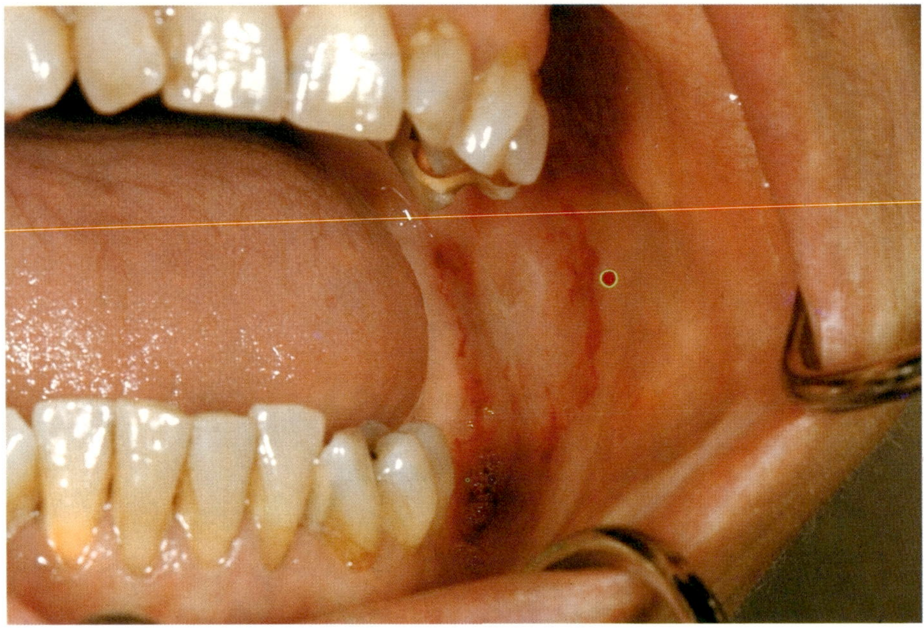

236

236 Dark-red discoloration in the mucosa of the pterygomandibular fold, with no ulceration or infiltration, immediately following spontaneous rupture of bullae in the mucosa. (Female aged 52, in good health; clinically, pemphigus vulgaris suspected)

237 Epithelium showing low-degree acanthosis and parakeratosis. Narrow spaces are discernible in the basal epithelium.

238 Greater magnification shows discrete dissolution of intercellular bridges between the basal and spindle cell layers.

239 A large space can be seen between basal and prickle cell layers (acantholysis). Normally developed, intact basal cells are clearly discernible, lined up like paving stones.

Clinical management

Excision biopsy should be done for histological examination. In this case (Figures **236** to **239**) pemphigus vulgaris was confirmed, and the patient referred to a dermatologist for further treatment.

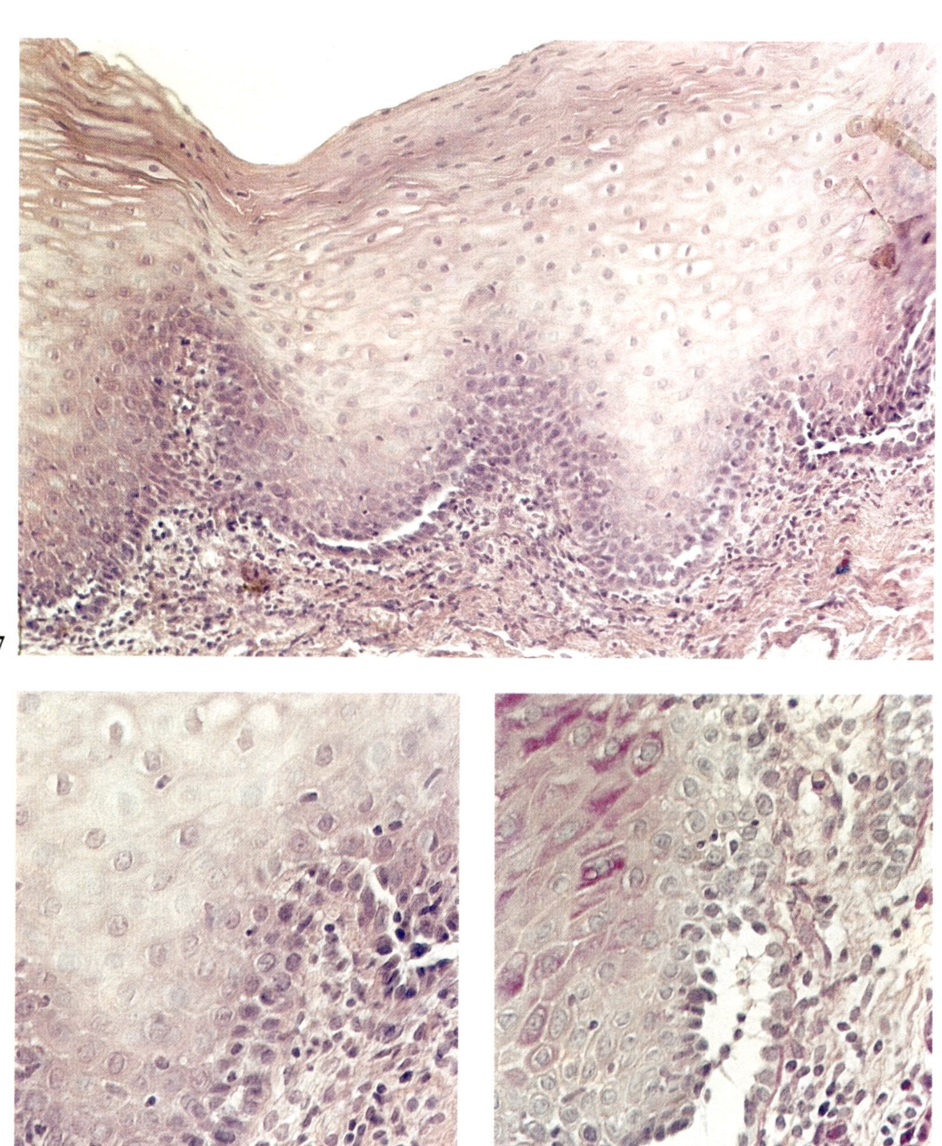

237

238

239

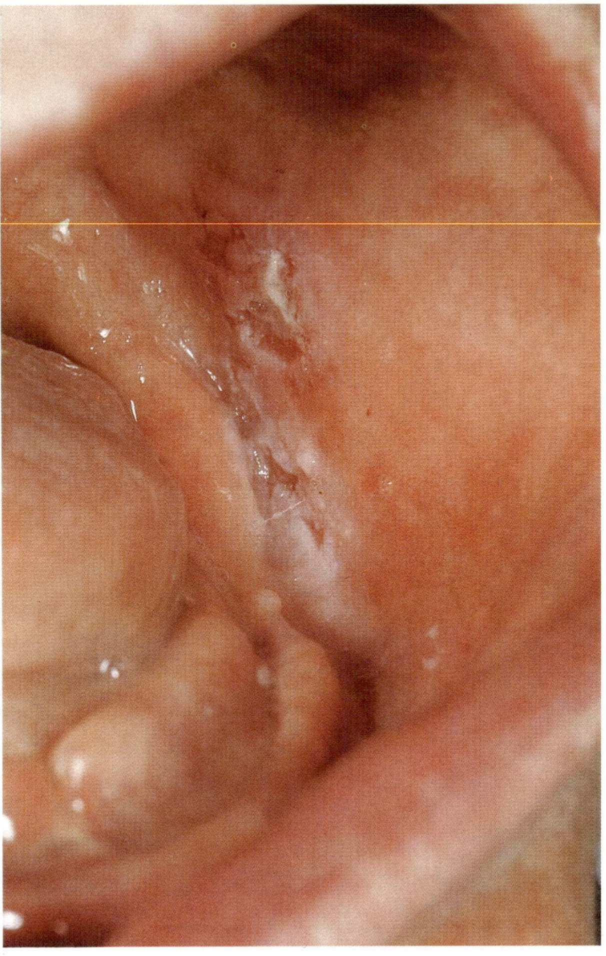

240

240 Several small, dark-red, partly confluent erosions in the oral mucosa, with no infiltration, but with whitish discoloration marginally in the buccoalveolar sulcus. (Female aged 70; highly suggestive of malignancy – erosive leukoplakia or early invasive carcinoma)

241 Epithelium showing acanthosis, hyperparakeratosis and extensive vesicles between basal and prickle cell layers. Subepithelial connective tissue is stained green. *(Masson–Goldner).*

242 Epithelial rete peg showing extensive vesicle formation between basal and prickle cell layers.

243 Extensive vesicles between basal and prickle cells. Basal cells are well maintained and show normal linkage with underlying stroma. The vesicle contains detached acantholytic prickle cells.

Clinical management

Admission to hospital for excision biopsy and histological examination of fast-frozen section. In this case (Figures **240** to **243**) no carcinoma was found, but pemphigus vulgaris was confirmed. The patient should be referred to a dermatologist for further treatment.

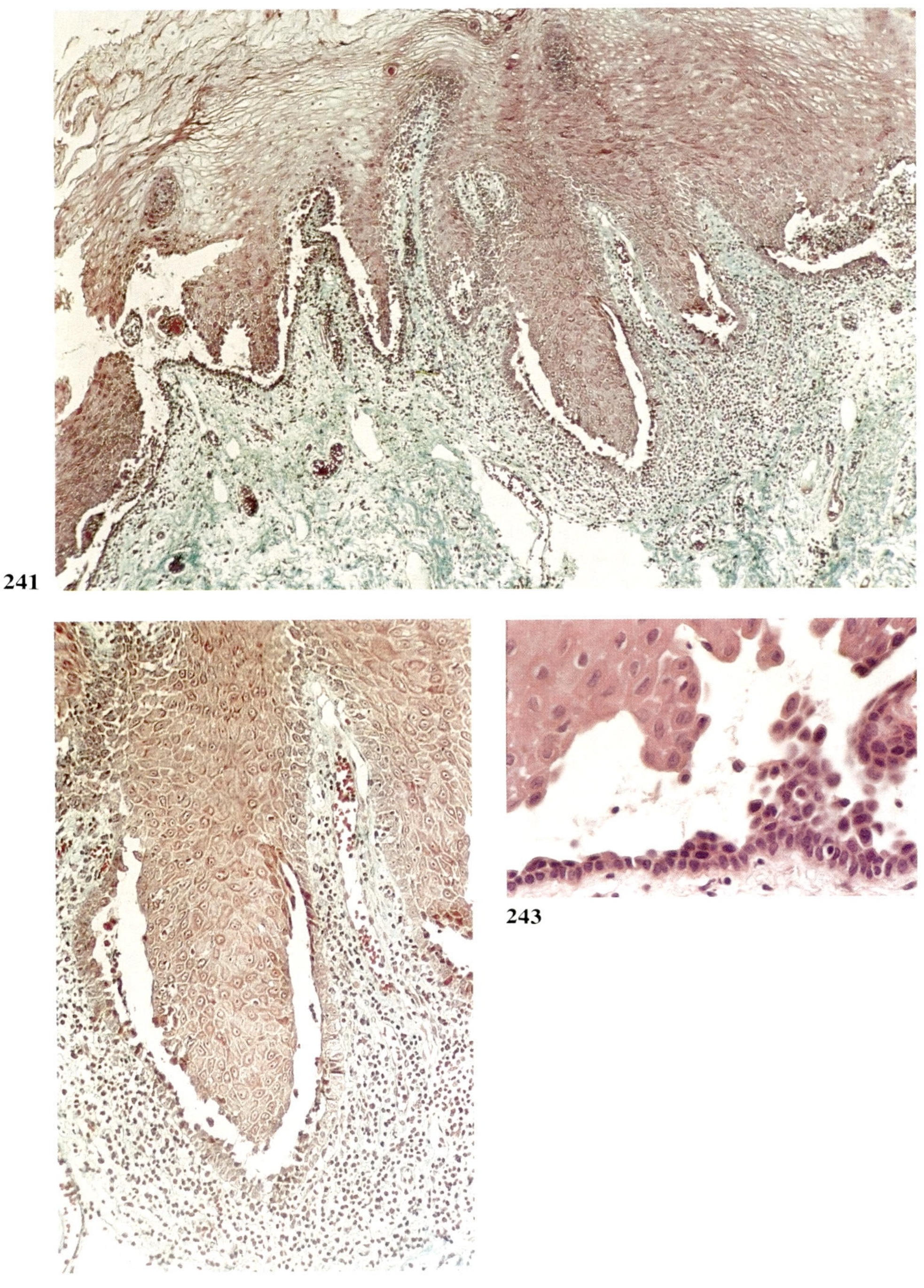

241

242

243

Dark pigmented patches (melanosis)

Dark patches or spots on the oral mucosa may be mentioned briefly in this context. Unless caused by foreign bodies (*e.g.* following injury in the course of dental treatment), they are usually the result of local accumulations of melanocytes and epithelial cells containing melanin, *i.e.* melanosis. The condition is a characteristic symptom of hypoadrenalism (Addison's disease). In Peutz–Jegher's syndrome the spots occur in association with intestinal polyps. A harmless melanosis of the oral mucosa is seen as a racial characteristic in coloured people, as are a wide variety of mixtures of whitish, red and dark areas in the mucosa.

Malignant melanoma is a rare condition of the oral mucosa. The superficial, spreading type starts as a dark spot. Rapid onset and growth should always be regarded as a warning signal in clinical practice.

With black hairy tongue, the filiform papillae are overgrown, and a particular mixed flora has become established in the area. This is a harmless change affecting the surface of the tongue.

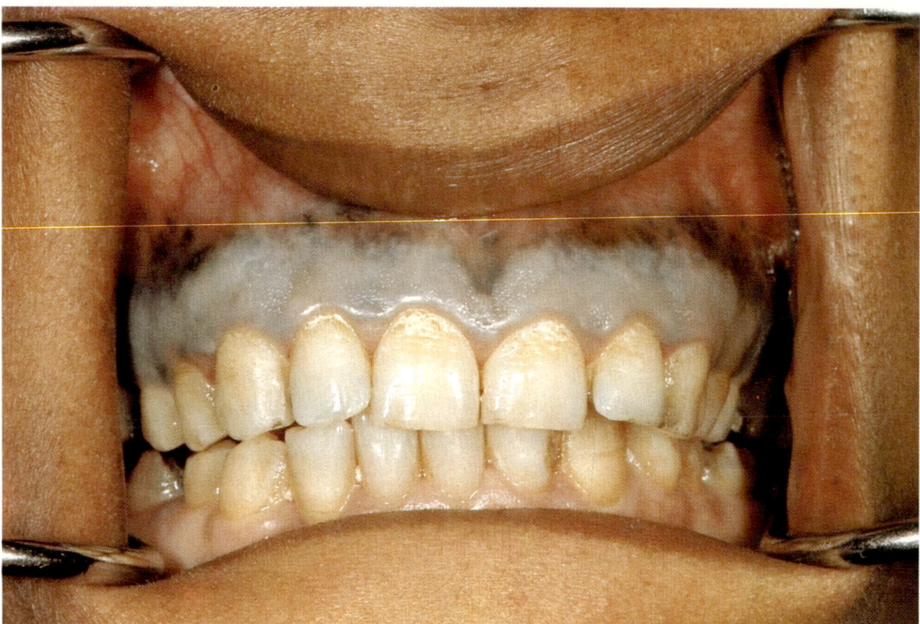

244

244 Bluish-white, non-hypertrophic discoloration of the whole gingiva propria in the upper jaw, with dark pigmentation in the margin. (Negress aged 30, in good health; clinically non-suspect)

245 Locostable mucosa from the gingiva showing normal structure, with deep epithelial and connective tissue interdigitation, normal epithelial stratification and dense collagen fibrous tissue subepithelially.

246 Clear view of connective tissue, with a narrow anucleated horny layer at the surface of the epithelium. The granular layer is not discernible under the light microscope. *(Masson–Goldner)*.

Clinical management

No treatment is required.

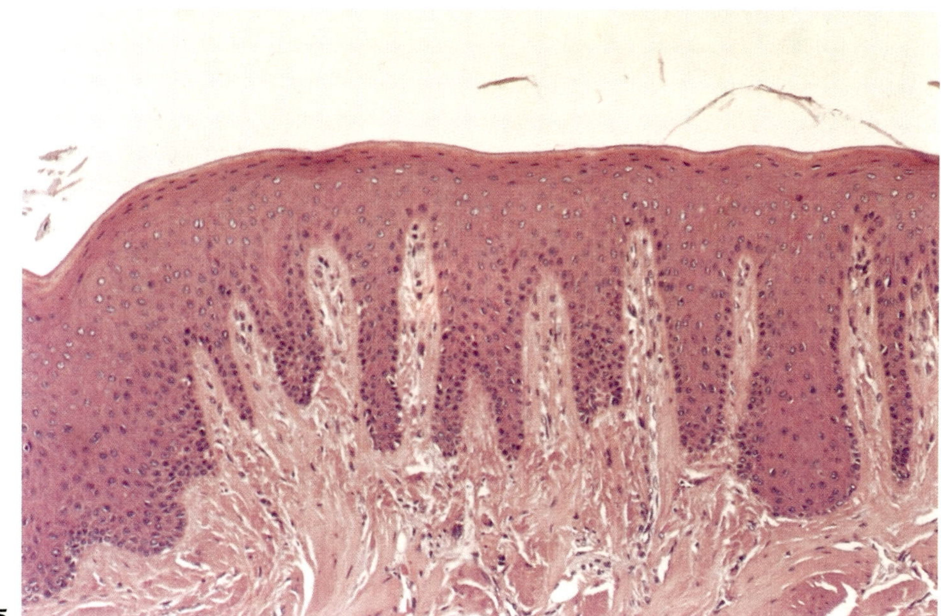

245

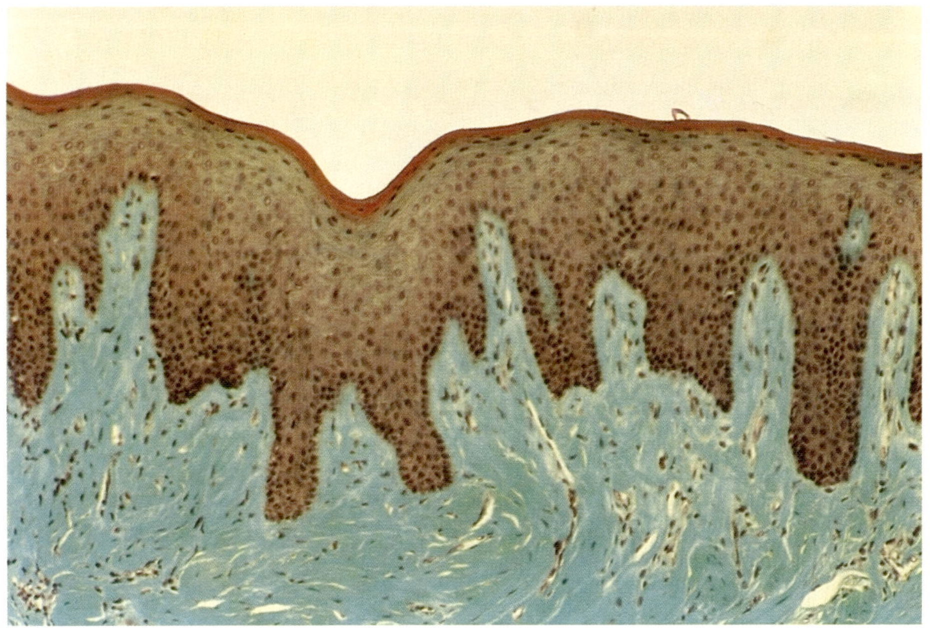

246

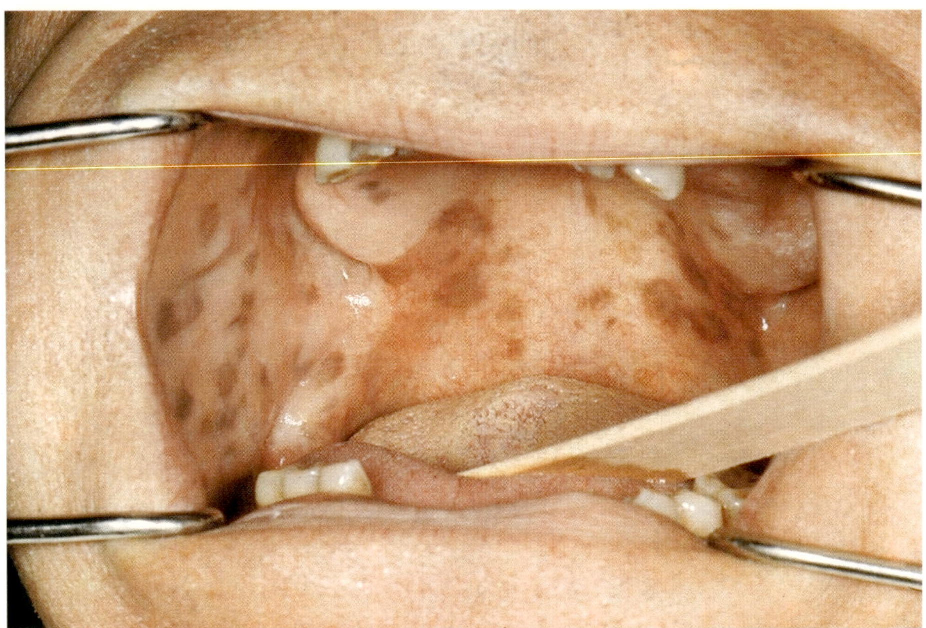

247

247 Planar, partly confluent brownish discoloration of the mucosa in the region of both cheeks and the palate, with no other changes. (Male aged 61; clinically, malignancy not suspected)

248 Epithelium from the palatal region showing normal stratification and well developed basal rete pegs. There is a brown pigmentation in the basal cell layer, and the subepithelial connective tissue contains many fibrous elements.

249 Narrow rete peg with marked brown pigmentation of cytoplasm in the basal cells.

Clinical management

Patient should be referred to medical specialist for exclusion of Addison's disease and Peutz–Jegher's syndrome. Local therapy is not required.

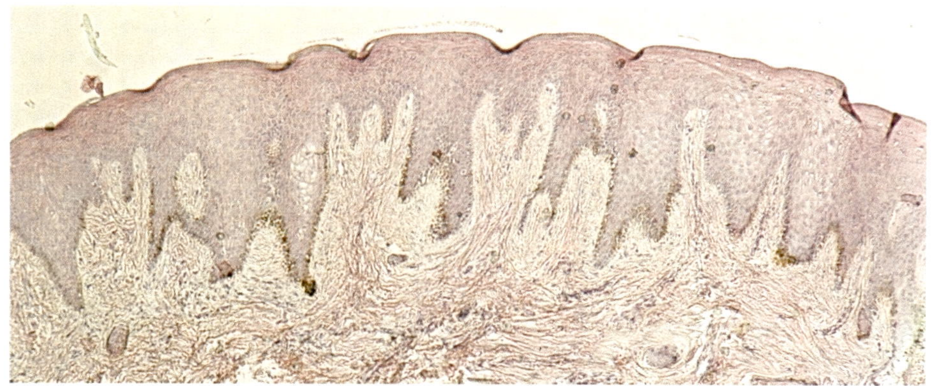

248

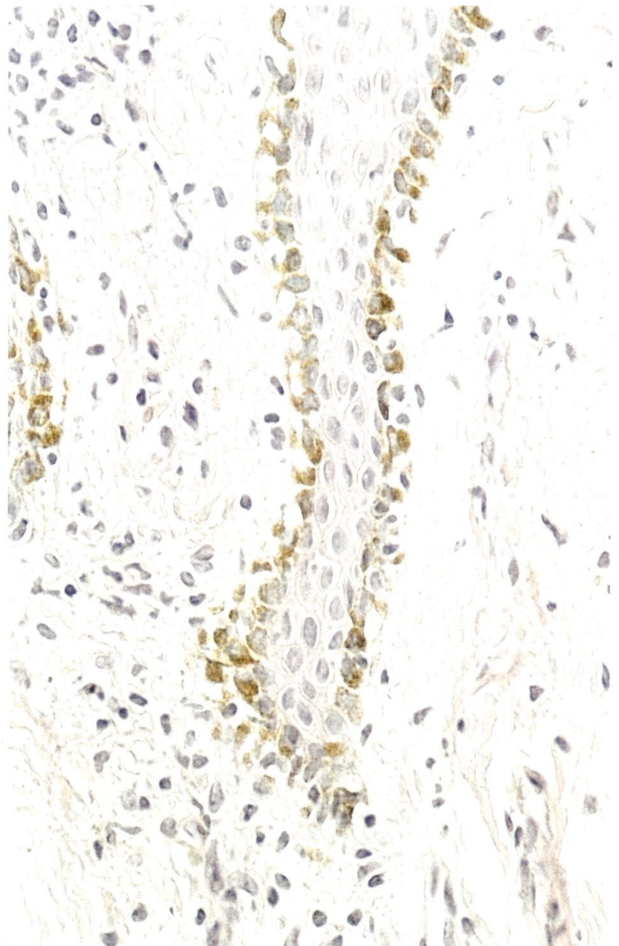

249

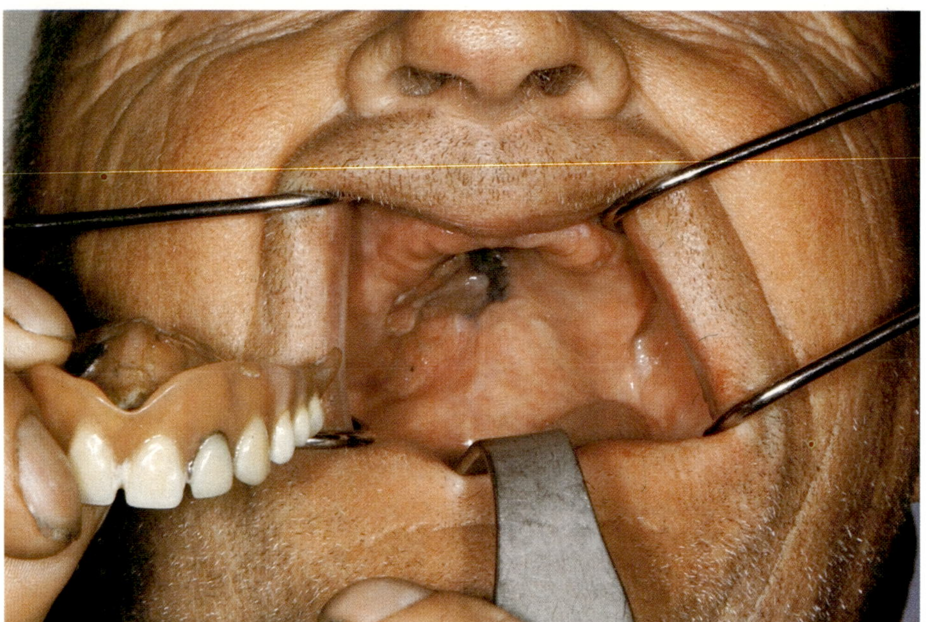

250

250 Nodular raised lesion in the mucosa of the anterior hard palate showing black pigmentation beneath full upper denture. (Male aged 63; clinically, malignant melanoma suspected)

251 Atrophic, orthokeratotic keratinising epithelium can be seen superficially. There is extensive proliferation of a polymorphic tumour in the basal epithelium and stroma and focal deposits of dense brown pigment in the cytoplasm.

252 Clearly atrophic epithelium with dense infiltration of polymorphic cells and large aggregates of brown melanin pigment.

Clinical management

Admission to hospital for resection of maxilla when fast-frozen section has confirmed the diagnosis. Follow-up oncological therapy is required.

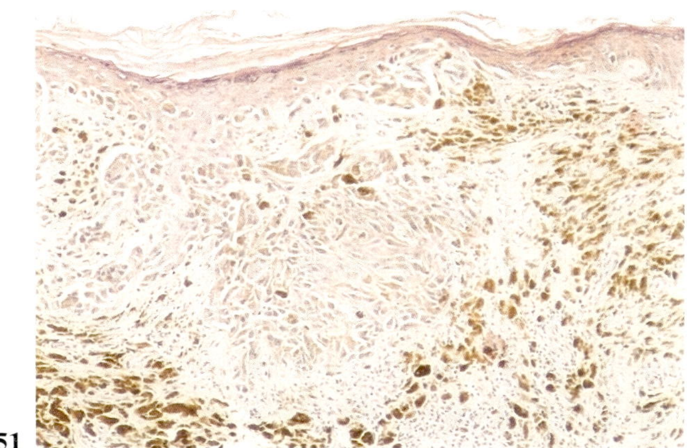
251

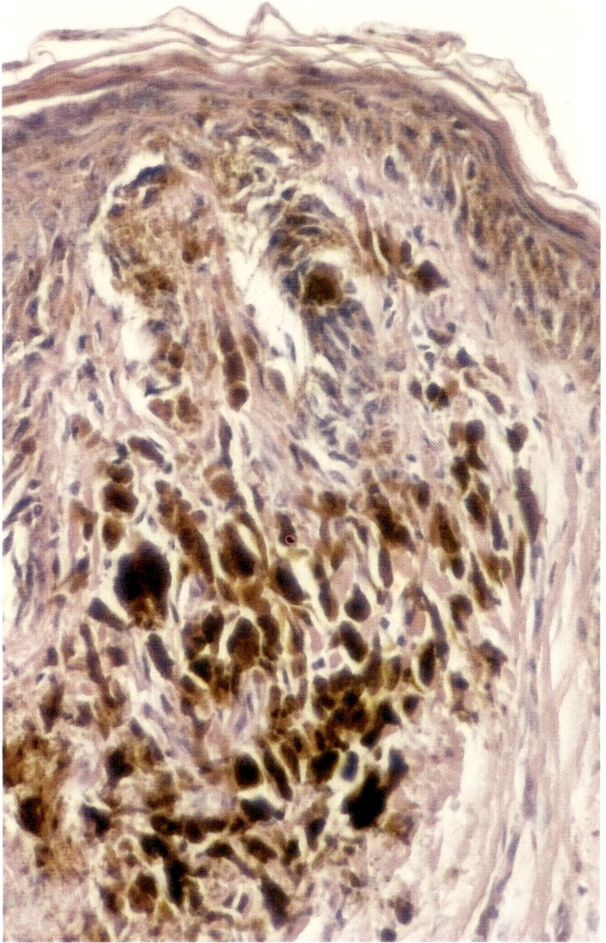
252

6 Bibliography

Bánóczy, J., L. Sugár: Longitudinal studies in oral leukoplakias. J. Oral Path. 1, 265–272 (1972)

Binnie, W. H.: Oral cancer. In: Oral mucosa in health and disease, p. 3–334. A. E. Dolby (Ed.). Blackwell Scientific Publications: Oxford, London, Edinburgh, Melbourne 1975

Burkhardt, A., G. Seifert: Morphologische Klassifikation der oralen Leukoplakien. Dtsch. med. Wschr. 102, 223–229 (1977)

Burkhardt, A., R. Maerker: Dysplasieklassifikation oraler Leukoplakien und Präkanzerosen. Bedeutung für Prognose und Therapie. Dtsch. Z. Mund-, Kiefer- u. Gesichts-Chir. 2, 199–205 (1978)

Burkhardt, A., R. Maerker, Th. Löning, G. Seifert: Dysplasieklassifikation oraler Leukoplakien und Präkanzerosen. Definition und praktische Anwendung. Dtsch. Z. Mund-, Kiefer- u. Gesichts-Chir. 2, 221–231 (1978)

Burkhardt, A.: Der Mundhöhlenkrebs und seine Vorstadien. Ultrastrukturelle und immunpathologische Aspekte. Veröffentlichungen aus der Pathologie Bd. 112. G. Fischer, Stuttgart–New York 1980

Cawson, R. A.: Chronic oral candidiasis and leukoplakia. Oral Surg. 22, 582–591 (1966)

Esser, E.: Therapie der intraoralen Leukoplakie. Dtsch. Z. Mund-, Kiefer- u. Gesichts-Chir. 3, 201–208 (1979)

Fasske, E., W. Hahn, K. Morgenroth, H. Themann: Die formale und kausale Genese der Leukoplakia oris. Z. Haut-Geschlechtskrh. 26, 339–347 (1959)

Gorlin, R. J., H. M. Goldman: Thoma's oral pathology. Mosby, St. Louis 1970

Graham, S., H. Dayal, T. Rohrer, M. Swanson, H. Sultz, D. Shedd, S. Fischman: Dentition, diet, tobacco, and alcohol in the epidemiology of oral cancer. J. Natl. Cancer Inst. 59, 1611 (1977)

Greither, A.: Die Einteilung der Leukoplakien. Arch. klin. exp. Dermat. 227, 798–802 (1966)

Hornstein, O. P.: Entzündliche und systemische Reaktionen in der Mundschleimhaut. Arch. Oto-Rhino-Laryng. 213, 287–331 (1976)

Horstein, O. P.: Orale Leukoplakien. I. Klassifikation, Differentialdiagnose, ätiologische Bedingungen der Kanzerisierung, Prognose. Dtsch. zahnärztl. Z. 32, 497–505 (1977)

Horstein, O. P., R. Gräßel, E. Schirner, H. Schell: Orale Candida-Besiedlung bei Leukoplakien und Karzinomen der Mundhöhle. Dtsch. med. Wschr. 104, 1033–1036 (1979)

Koch, H.: Karzinome der Mundhöhle. Westdeutscher Verlag, Opladen 1974

Kramer, I. R. H.: Precancerous conditions of the oral mucosa. Ann. Roy. Coll. Surg. Engl. 45, 340–356 (1969)

Kramer, I. R. H.: Carcinoma-in-situ of the oral mucosa. Int. Dent. J. 23, 94–99 (1973)

Lehner, T.: Immunopathology of oral leukoplakia. Brit. J. Cancer 24, 442–446 (1970)

Löning, Th., A. Burkhardt, G. Seifert, J.-O. Gebbers: Zur Typisierung der Immunglobuline in oralen Leukoplakien und Karzinomen. Dtsch. Z. Mund-, Kiefer- u. Gesichts-Chir. 1, 168–177 (1977)

Löning, Th., A. Burkhardt: Häufigkeit von Epitheldysplasien der Mundschleimhaut. Histologische Studie an 150 Obduktionsfällen. Dtsch. Z. Mund-, Kiefer- u. Gesichts-Chir. 2, 232–242 (1978)

MacDonald, D. G.: Premalignant lesions of oral epithelium. In: Oral mucosa in health and disease, p. 335–369. A. E. Dolby (Ed.). Blackwell Scientific Publications, Oxford, London, Edinburgh, Melbourne 1975

Maerker, R., A. Burkhardt: Klinik oraler Leukoplakien und Präkanzerosen. Retrospektive Studie an 200 Patienten. Dtsch. Z. Mund-, Kiefer- u. Gesichts-Chir. 2, 206–220 (1978)

Mashberg, A.: Erythroplasia – earliest sign of asymptomatic oral cancer. J. Am. Dent. Ass. 96, 615–620 (1978)

Mehta, F. S., D. K. Daftary, B. C. Shroff, L. D. Sangvi: Clinical and histologic study of oral leukoplakia in relation to habits. Oral Surg. 28, 372–388 (1969)

Pape, H. D.: Die Früherkennung der malignen Mundschleimhauttumoren unter besonderer Berücksichtigung der exfoliativen Zytologie. Carl Hanser, München 1972

Pindborg, J. J., G. Renstrup, H. E. Poulsen, S. Silverman: Studies in oral leukoplakia. V. Clinical and histological signs of malignancy. Acta Odont. Scand. 21, 407–414 (1963)

Pindborg, J. J., O. Jolst, G. Renstrup, B. Roed-Petersen: Studies in oral leukoplakia: a preliminary report on the period prevalence of malignant transformation in leukoplakia based on a follow-up study of 248 patients. J. Am. Dent. Ass. 76, 767–771 (1968)

Pindborg, J. J.: Atlas der Erkrankungen der Mundschleimhaut. Carl Hanser, München 1969

Pindborg, J. J.: Oral cancer and precancer. John Wright & Sons, Bristol 1980

Pogrel, M. A.: Sublingual keratosis and malignant transformation. J. Oral Pathol. 8, 176–178 (1979)

Roed-Petersen, B.: Cancer development in oral leukoplakia. Follow-up of 331 patients. J. Dent. Res. 50, 711 (1971)

Roed-Petersen, B., P. C. Gupta, J. J. Pindborg, B. Singh: Association between oral leukoplakia and sex, age, and tobacco habits. Bull. WHO 47, 13–19 (1972)

Schuermann, H., A. Greither, O. Hornstein: Krankheiten der Mundschleimhaut und der Lippen. Verlag Urban & Schwarzenberg, München–Berlin–Wien 1966

Schwimmer, E.: Die idiopathischen Schleimhautplaques der Mundhöhle (Leucoplakia buccalis). Arch. Dermat. Syph. 9, 511–570 (1877)

Seifert, G.: Mundhöhle, Mundspeicheldrüsen, Tonsillen und Rachen. In: Spezielle pathologische Anatomie, Bd. 1. Doerr, Uehlinger, Seifert (Eds.). J. Springer, Berlin–Heidelberg–New York 1966

Seifert, G., A. Burkhardt: Neuere morphologische Gesichtspunkte bei malignen Tumoren der Mundschleimhaut. Dtsch. Med. Wschr. 102, 1596–1601 (1977)

Seifert, G., M. Vossmeyer: Glossitis rhombica mediana (Brocq). Pathologisch-anatomische Analyse von 28 Fällen. Dtsch. Z. Mund-, Kiefer- u. Gesichts-Chir. 2, 162–170 (1978)

Seifert, G., A. Burkhardt: Orale Krebsvorstadien. Oral precancer. Verh. Dtsch. Ges. Path. 63, 74–96 (1979)

Shafer, W. G., C. A. Waldron: A clinical and histopathologic study of oral leukoplakia. Surg. Gynec. Obstet. 112, 411–420 (1961)

Shafer, W. G.: Oral carcinoma in situ. Oral Surg. 39, 227–238 (1975)

Shklar, G.: The precancerous oral lesion. Oral Surg. 20, 58–70 (1965)

Smith, C. J.: Global epidemiology and aetiology of oral cancer. Int. Dent. J. 23, 82–93 (1973)

Spiessl, B.: Plattenepithelkarzinom der Mundhöhle. Grundlagen der Behandlung. G. Thieme, Stuttgart 1966

Spiessl, B., H.-J. Metz: Differentialdiagnose und Behandlung der Leukoplakie. Dtsch. Zahn-, Mund-u.Kieferheilk. 48, 11–21 (1967)

Strassburg, M., G. Knolle: Farbatlas der Mundschleimhauterkrankungen. Die Quintessenz, Berlin 1973

Tyldesley, W. R.: A Colour Atlas of Oral Medicine, Wolfe Medical Publications, London 1978

Waldron, C. A., W. G. Shafer: Leukoplakia revisited. A clinico-pathologic study of 3256 oral leukoplakias. Cancer 36, 1386–1392 (1975)

WHO Collaborating Centre for oral precancerous lesions. Definition of leukoplakia and related lesions: an aid to studies on oral precancer. Oral Surg. 46, 518–539 (1978)

Wilsch, L., O. P. Hornstein, H. Brüning, V. Schwipper, F. Lösel, A. Schönberger, W. Gunselmann, H. Prestele: Orale Leukoplakien. II. Ergebnisse einer 1-jährigen poliklinischen Pilotstudie. Dtsch. zahnärztl. Z. 33, 132–142 (1978)

Index

References are to page numbers

Acantholysis, in pemphigus vulgaris, 171, 172
Acanthosis, 28 (table), 138
- in leukoplakia, 36,40,44
- in lichen planus, 166, 168
- in median rhomboid glossitis, 132
- in morsicatio buccarum, 152
- in pemphigus vulgaris, 171, 174
- in white spong naevus, 114, 116
Ackermann's tumour, 82
Addison's disease, 177, 180
Alcohol, 24 (table)
Apthous ulcers, 141, 148
Attachment plaques, 13

Basal cells, 18
- hyperplasia of, 28 (table), 29
- loss of polarity, 28 (table), 29
- in pemphigus vulgaris, 171, 172
Basal membrane, 18
- in leukoplakia, 29, 30, 31, 44, 52, 73
Benzol, 24 (table)
Betel nut chewing, 9, 24 (table), 151
Black hairy tongue, 177
Bleomycin, 83
Bouin's solution, 28–9

Candida albicans, 24 (table), 26
- in denture wearers, 26
- and leukoplakia, 34
- in median rhomboid glossitis, 129
Carcinoma of mouth, anaplasia grading, 82
- atypia grading, 82
- early stages, 81–111
- - clinical features, 81
- - histopathology, 81–2
- - therapy, 83
- grading I–IV, 82
- incidence, 5, 9
Carcinoma dissimulans, 81
Carcinoma *in situ*, 65, 76, 78
- biopsies over 10 years, 34 (table)
- characteristics, 33 (table), 33–4
- clinical progress of patients, 35
Cellular polymorphism, epithelial, 28 (table)
Cheek-biting, 24 (table), 151, 152
Cheek pouch, mucosal changes in, 151, 154–5
Cheilitis, 135
Chesa stain, 28, 100
Coca leaf chewing, 9, 151
Collagen fibrous tissue, with granulomata, 138
Connective tissue papillae, 13 (table), 14

Dentures, irritation from, 24 (table), 26
Desmosomes, 13
Diabetes mellitus, 24 (table)
Differential diagnosis, 113–83
Discoid lupus erythematosus, 113 (table), 113
Dissimulating cancers, 81
Dyskeratosis, 28 (table), 29, 32, 62
Dysplasia, 5, 10, 28–9
- biopsy material, 34 (table)
- characteristics, 28 (table), 29, 33 (table)
- classifications, prognosis and treatment relationships, 34, 80 (table)
Dysplastic epithelial atrophy, 13

Elastoid degeneration of connective tissue, 60
Endophytic cone, 104
Epithelial cone, 146
Epithelial dysplasia, characteristics, 28 (table), 29
Epithelial hyperplasia, characteristics, 28 (table)
Epithelial-mesenchymal interface, 18
- in leukoplakia, 31
Epithelial ridges, normal, 114
Epithelium, endophytic, 65, 67, 68, 70
- exophytic, 50, 54
Epithelium, stratified, 13
- abnormal, 28 (table), 29
- basal layer, 13 (table), 13, 16, 18
- - in leukoplakia, 38, 40, 42, 46, 48, 54, 58, 62, 65
-granular layer, 13 (table), 13
- - in leukoplakia, 44, 46
- horny layer, 13 (table), 13, 21
- - in leukoplakia, 36, 38, 40, 42, 44, 46
- orthokeratosis (anucleate), 13 (table), 13, 17, 28 (table), 38
- parakeratosis (nucleate), 13, 13 (table), 21, 28 (table)
- - in leukoplakia, 40, 42
- prickle cell layer, *see* Prickle cells
- regeneration of, 146
- in smoker's palate, 120
- spinous layer (stratum spinosum), 13, 16
- - in leukoplakia, 32
- in white sponge naevus, 114, 116
Erosion, inflammatory, 144, 146
Erythema multiforme, 113 (table)
Erythroplakia, 13, 24
- biopsy, 26, 27–8
- classification, 32
- clinical aspects, 24–6
- diagnosis, 26–7

Fordyce spots, 157, 158
Fibromas, pedunculate, 52
Fungal hyphae, 70

Galvanic irritation, 24 (table)
Geographic tongue, 113 (table), 125–7
Glossitis, granulomatous, 135
- syphilitic, 113
Glossitis migrans, 113 (table), 125–7
Glossitis rhombica mediana, 113 (table), 129–33
Glycogen, intracellular, in leukoplakia, 36, 42
Granulomata, 138

Haematoxylin and eosin stain, 28
Hereditary factors, 24 (table)
Herpes virus, 24 (table)
Heterotopic sebaceous glands, 157, 158
Histological assessment and dysplasia classification, 28–34
Histological examination, 27–8
Hormonal factors, 24 (table)
Horned pearl, 65
Horny layer, superficial, 21
Hyperkeratosis, 13, 28 (table)
- in pemphigus vulgaris, 174
Hyperorthokeratosis, in leukoplakia, 46, 48, 56
Hyperparakeratosis, in leukoplakia, 48, 52, 58, 68
- in lichen planus, 166, 168
- in morsicatio buccarum, 152
- in white sponge naevus, 114, 116
Hypoadrenalism, 177

Immunocompetent cells, 14
Immunological reactions, 5
Intercellular bridges, dissolution of, in pemphigus vulgaris, 172
Intercellular spaces, 32
Interepithelial cells, increase of, 32
Intra-epithelial suprabasal vesicles, in pemphigus vulgaris, 171
Iron deficiency, 24 (table)

Keratin, staining of, 28, 100
- stratified lamellae of, 100
Keratinisation, 13, 16, 100, 110
- organoid, 65
Keratin pools, 36

Lamina propria, 13 (table)
Lead, 24 (table)
Leukocytes, 14
Leukoedema, 28 (table), 36
Leukokeratosis nicotinica palati, 23, 113 (table), 119–23
Leukoplakia, 9–10, 13, 23–80
- aetiological classification, 23–4
- aetiological factors, 24
- age of patient, 26
- basement membrane in, 29, 30, 31, 44, 52, 73
- biopsy, 26, 27–8
- classification by dysplasia, 28–34
- clinical aspects, 24–6, 25 (table)
- clinical management, 80 (tables)
- clinical prognosis with differing degrees of dysplasia, 34, 35 (tables)
- diagnosis, 26–7
- dysplasia and, 29, 33–4
- - high degree of, 33 (table), 33–4, 34 (table), 35
- - low degree of, 29, 33 (table), 34, 35
- - moderate degree of, 33, 33 (table), 34 (table), 35
- ebb-tide, 46
- endogenous irritative, 23
- erosive, 25–6, 25 (table)
- exogenous irritative, 23
- harmless, 29
- hereditary, 23
- histological assessment, 28–34
- hyperorthokeratosis in, 46, 48, 56
- hyperparaketatosis in, 48, 52, 58, 68
- idiopathic, 23
- localisation of, 26
- patchy, 26
- prognosis, 26
- sex distribution, 26
- simple, 24, 25 (tables)
- tonofibrils in, 29, 30, 31, 32
- verrucous, 24–5, 25 (tables)
Leukoplakia carcinomata, 64, 81
Lichen planus, 23, 113 (table), 113, 161–9
- epithelium in, 164, 166, 168
- hyperparakeratosis in, 166, 168
- whitish changes in mucosa, 168
Lingua geographica, 113 (table), 125–7
Lip, carcinoma of, 106, 108
Liver disease, 24 (table)
Lymphocytes, subepithelial, increase of, 29

Malignant melanoma, 177, 182
Malnutrition, 24 (table)
Masson-Goldner stain, 17, 28, 40, 54, 86, 126, 132, 174, 178
Median rhomboid glossitis, 113 (table), 129–33
- mucosal discolouration in, 132
Melanosis, 177–83
Melkersson-Rosenthal syndrome, 135
Mercury, 24 (table)
Mitosis, increase rate of, 28 (table), 29
Morsicatio buccarum, 24 (table), 151, 152
- hyperparakeratosis in, 152
Mucosa, oral, 13–21
- dark patches (spots) on, 177–83
- discoloured lesions in leukoplakia, 36, 38, 40, 44, 46, 48, 50, 52, 58, 72
- early cancer of, 84, 86, 88, 90, 92, 94, 96, 110
- erosive lesions of, 64, 66, 68
- - in pipe smokers, 60, 62, 64
- histological structure, 13
- in lichen planus, 164
- locolabile, 13
- locostabile, 13, 178
- non-malignant ulceration, 141–9
- and oral habits, 151–5
- in pemphigus vulgaris, 174
- pigmentation of, 178, 180, 182
- punctate erosion of, 154
- red lesions, 76, 78
- in smoker's palate, 120, 122
- starting point of oral cancer, 9
- white changes, inflammatory, 135–9
- whitish verrucous change in, 136
Muscularis mucosae, 14

Naevus spongiosus albus mucosae, *see* White sponge naevus
Nodular stroma reaction, 73

Oral habits, 9, 24 (table), 151–5
Orthokeratosis, 13, 28 (table), 58, 164

Palate, cancer of, 98, 102, 104
– normal mucosa, 17
Papillomatous exophytic epithelium, 50
Parakeratosis, 13, 28 (table), 138
– in pemphigus vulgaris, 172
– in white sponge naevus, 114
Pemphigus vulgaris, 113 (table), 171–5
– intercellular bridges dissolved in, 172
– intra-epithelial suprabasal vesicles in, 171
Periodic-acid-Schiff stain (PAS), 28, 34, 42, 65, 70, 73, 78, 116, 152
Periodontium, inflamed, erosion associated, 144
Peutz-Jegher syndrome, 177, 180
Plasma cells, increase of, 29
Plasma membranes, 21
Precancerous lesions, 23–80
– aetiological factors, 24 (table)
Preneoplasms, multiple, 5
Prickle cells, 13 (table), 13, 18, 21, 30, 31, 32
– ballooning of, 152
– in leukoplakia, 30, 31, 32, 36, 38, 40, 42, 48, 60, 70
– in lichen planus, 168
– oedematous, 152
– in white sponge naevus, 116
Psoriasis, 113 (table)

Rete pegs, 13 (table), 14, 16, 17
– in leukoplakia, 40, 46, 50, 52, 54, 56, 67, 72, 74
– in median rhomboid glossitis, 130, 132
– in pemphigus vulgaris, 174
– saw-toothed, in lichen planus, 162, 164, 166
– in smoker's palate, 122
– in white sponge naevus, 116
Russell bodies, 67, 78

Sebaceous glands, heterotopic, 157, 158
Seromucous glands, with lymphocytic infiltration around, 142
Smoker's palate, 23, 113 (table), 119–23
– squamous epithelium of glandular duct, 120, 122
Smoking, 9, 151
Spices, abuse of, 151
Spindle cell carcinoma, 82
Spongiosis, 28 (table)
Spongy epithelium, 136
Squamous epithelium of glandular duct, in smoker's palate, 120, 122
Stains, histological, 28, 34
– *see also individual stains*
Stars (intercellular spaces), 32
Stroma reaction, 32
Subepithelial connective tissue, 14
Subepithelial stroma inflammatory reaction, in lichen planus, 166
Submucous fibrosis, 13
Syphilis, 24 (table), 142

Tobacco, abuse of, 9, 24 (table), 151
– chewing, 9, 151
Tongue, cancer of, 98
– discolouration of mucosa, 42, 54, 56, 74
– normal mucosa, 15
– markings on, in lichen planus, 166
– white-grey striated nodular lesions on, 138
Tonofibrils, 13, 18
– in leukoplakia, 29, 30, 31, 32

Ulcerative epithelial defect, 136

Verrucous carcinoma, 82, 104, 106
Vesicles beteen basal and prickle cells, in pemphigus vulgaris, 174
Viral focal epithelial hyperplasia, 113 (table)

White sponge naevus, 113 (table), 113–14, 116
– hyperparakeratosis in, 114, 116
– rete pegs in, 114
– mucosal discolouration in, 113, 114, 116
World Health Organisation, Cancer Unit, 23